I0441411

Dances with my Father

By Wendy Alexander

Contents

Prologue

The Collins dictionary defines cancer as: 'a serious disease resulting from a malignant growth or tumour caused by abnormal and excessive cell division.'

I don't care how it's defined; I only know I don't like it. My reaction is similar to my daughter's, whose response was 'I hate cancer, mummy,' when she found out her grandpa had prostate cancer.

Up until dad's cancer diagnosis, our family's experience with the disease was secondary — through the experiences of friends, work colleagues and extended family. Now it's shown up and entered our family sanctuary going straight for our captain and knocking the wind from our sails. We weren't prepared for this. I don't know that anyone's ever prepared. Despite the fact that cancer appears to be the dominating disease of this century, I think every one hopes they or their loved ones will be spared. I know I did.

But it's here now and I realised that all my moaning, groaning or asking 'why?' will not change that. The only positive (if it can be viewed as such) is that it's a disease that forces one to focus on the possibility of death while trying to get as much life out of life as one can.

And I discovered one important thing during my first weeks of processing my feelings about cancer and its intrusion into dad's life. I wasn't going to wait until a final curtain call to pay tribute to the person who has most influenced my life. Eulogies are wonderful but wasted on the dead. Words of gratitude and tribute should be expressed often and especially while our loved ones are still here.

<u>Dances with my father</u>
I danced my first dance with you
Through the weaving of words
As stories of fantasy and witches brew
And princes, paupers and ghastly cowards
Captured my mind and delighted my heart

Every dance since, no matter the step
Light with joy, heavy with woe
Or simply another wandering sidestep
Caught in the choices of life's crossbow
Are the dances with my father I won't forget.

Dance with my Father

If I could get another chance,
another walk, another dance with him
I'd play a song that would never, ever end
How I'd love, love, love
To dance with my father again.

('Dance with my father' — *Luther Van Dross*)

I don't imagine I'll forget 6 May 2010 anytime soon — the day that dreaded disease cancer found its way into our family. I'm not a stranger to the disease — who is these days? There's hardly a person I've met who hasn't had to confront it at one time or another. Until now it was something I experienced through someone else's journey, mostly friends or work colleagues. I often wondered if it would ever come knocking on my family door, I never expected it to be my dad though. At sixty eight years of age, he's one of the healthiest people I know. He cycles most days, and takes daily walks for forty-five minutes to an hour, regularly visits the spa and sauna and eats very well (probably more than he should, but dad's had a love affair with food for as long as I can remember). Fortunately for him, mum is the best cook on this planet (or so my daughter proclaims) and has by and large put healthy food on his plate every day. She's not been able to convince him to reduce his portions, but since he does so much exercise, we never really worried too much about his health. We'd often tease dad that he only exercised so much so he could eat more. He'd never deny it; only grin in amusement.

When my youngest sister called me at work to tell me dad had been diagnosed with prostate cancer, I could hear my mind saying 'NO, absolutely no way!' I could feel my spirit shift into denial. Yet I knew it was true. I heard the raspy sound of her voice and the suppressed tears behind her words. I also knew dad had had an appointment with the urologist that day.

Time ground to a halt, as did my movements. I walked to the nearest quiet room in the office and just sat - for ten minutes. I can't remember now what thoughts ran through my head or if any did at all. I just know I wasn't ready to take that news in. I wanted to punch 'cancer' on the nose and slam our family door hard in its face. It had been hovering closer to the perimeters of my immediate family. I'd lost a girlfriend to breast cancer two years ago. Rihab was only two years older than me and had battled for about five years before she died in May 2008. She creeps into my mind often, especially when I hear music she used to love or stumble across passages or books she used to read. In May 2010, I started re-reading *The Prophet* by Kahlil Gibran — one of her favourites. She was a constant pulse in my memory.

Another dear friend, who has her birthday in May — has just come through lymphoma. 'Remission' was the result of months of chemo, radiation and a buffet of pills to combat the side effects. She wanted to hear 'cure", but the tumour is still there, just dormant. A year ago, also in May, another friend lost her mother to cancer. Now, the month of May, the month we celebrate my mum's birthday and Mother's day, isn't a month of joy as it's been in the past. Now it feels overshadowed by loss, sadness and fear.

Once I emerged from my quiet meeting room I sought out my boss. I knew I was zombie-like so figured I'd need to let someone know so my colleagues wouldn't speculate about my mental health. And if anyone would understand it would be him. He too has been through cancer having spent the last two years fighting lymphoma. His support, advice and understanding were exactly what I needed. And he warned me there was a gamut of emotions still to come and to be prepared for them to hit me and my family when we least expected it.

I nodded as if understanding, but really it was a reflex. I was still shocked and numbed by the news. But I had a repetitive flashing thought — I needed and wanted to speak with my dad, but I knew calling him from work was not the way to go. I had no idea how I'd be when I actually heard his voice. Thankfully, I only had a few minutes of my working day left so I passed that hiding in the rest room, taking deep breaths.

I had arranged, weeks earlier, to stay over at my boyfriend's place, a stone's throw from the city. My daughter was away on school camp and I had an early morning start at a three-day property conference in the city. As I drove through the city to pick him up I reminded myself to not say anything about dad until we were safely ensconced in his apartment. I wasn't sure I'd be able to tell him without bursting into tears and as I was navigating heavy city traffic, I needed my wits about me. But the heart doesn't always do what the mind commands. He'd barely gotten into the car when I blurted the news. And I didn't cry.

In fact it felt like someone else was speaking — my voice sounded emotionless and factual. I may as well have been telling him which footy team was sitting at the top of the league. But I know I was distracted and definitely half present as we ate Vietnamese food for dinner. And I kept repeating that I wanted to talk to my dad.

When I finally made the call to my parents' home the first thing I heard in the background was laughter. Dad was still laughing when he said 'hello' and he shared that he, mum and my siblings were just talking and laughing about the fact that he wouldn't have to worry about losing his hair since he was already bald. I can't say I was surprised to hear him say that. Our family has approached most things with a sense of humour over the years and I suppose this wasn't going to be any different. But somewhere in the deepest part of me I could feel something else lurking and sooner or later it would surface.

I asked dad if he wanted me to cancel my conference and be around on the weekend. His answer, true to form, was an emphatic 'No. Life goes on, so why would you want to cancel your conference?' he said. He's a tough old bugger and has fought the good fight in every challenging situation in his life. He was going to do nothing less in confronting his cancer. I did wonder though if he was inwardly scared. Dad and I are very similar in our approach to life. We take the position of strength when anything difficult or unexpected crosses our path; not ones to fall apart easily.

That night, though, I was scared. I wasn't ready to face the mortality of my father. Even though I knew if anyone had a fighting chance at beating this disease, it was my dad. The mental images I had of cancer — the loss of energy, the wasting away, the nausea and vomiting, the fear I'd seen in the eyes of cancer victims and their families — scared me. I was scared my dad — invincible in my eyes since I was a mere tot —would be reduced to a fraction of the strong, physical being I'd come to count on. And, truth be told, I'd thought mum might one day be the person who battled a terminal illness since she's always had health challenges and has been on various medications for years. My father has not had to take any for his entire sixty-eight years; he only takes a natural remedy called glucosamine and a fish oil capsule every day. How in the world could this be happening to him?

Long after my boyfriend was snoring next to me, I lay awake. Two conflicting ideas ran through me — 'there's a reason for everything' and 'why?'

When I pray I usually talk to angels. In my mind I muttered a hundred 'whys' and would try to comfort myself with 'I need to trust the angels, there's a reason for everything.' I can tell you now, — though I meditate, commune with God in nature, pray each day to angels — on that day, the 'whys' were winning out. I wasn't able to do anything but ask how this would affect my loved ones, or me.

I eventually fell asleep, for about two hours. I woke with another thought and sat bolt upright in bed. This couldn't be happening because I hadn't yet danced with my father at my wedding. At forty-three, I have yet to walk up the aisle. The longest relationship I've had —just over eight years — was with my daughter's father. I've had a few others before and after him, but none have led to marriage. I'm in a relationship now and it's great. (I guess one does gain some wisdom by the time we reach our forties.) But, even though we've known each other for a long time, the romantic partnership is new and so there's been no talk of marriage and long-term future.

Still, I dream of marrying some day. In and amongst the fantasies of my wedding day has always been an image of me dancing with my dad. When I first heard Luther Van Dross' song 'Dance with my father' I made a mental note then that would be the song I'd want to dance to, with my dad, on my wedding day.

As I thought about the possibility of that not happening, the first silent tears ran down my cheeks since I'd heard the diagnosis of prostate cancer.

Why can't the English

Why can't the English teach their children how to speak?
This verbal class distinction, by now,
Should be antique. If you spoke as she does, sir,
Instead of the way you do,
Why, you might be selling flowers, too!

(*'*Why can't the English' from *My Fair Lady)*

My conversations with my angels that morning were far from angelic. I even used a few four-letter curse words, wondering why this was happening to me. Oh yes. I'd already forgotten that it was really happening to dad. While I cried quietly to myself, I did wonder about the self-indulgent nature of human beings. I was mad; not only about dad's mortality, but because there's some unfinished business he's supposed to experience with me.

Another deep desire I have is for my father to see my books published and in bookstores. I've been steadily working on a series of writing projects and pursuing publication of some of these. From all accounts of professional writers this is a long and tedious process and many writing pieces never make it to publication because people give up long before their tenth rejection. Like my dad, I'm not a quitter, but now there's a sense of urgency for me to realise this dream.

I felt like punching my pillow, but knew it would wake my boyfriend. As selfish as I felt in that moment, I wasn't selfish enough to disturb the peaceful sleep of a loved one. He at least looked a lot more angelic than I felt even though I was the one talking to angels.

As I thought about wanting dad to see my novels published and in bookstores, a bubble of laughter rose in me. It shed a welcome light on my dark and angry thoughts like the first rays of dawn chases away the night. My boss had been right — that gamut of emotions was showing up and it hadn't yet been twenty-four hours since dad's diagnosis.

It was dad who first ignited my passion for literature and writing so many years ago. It was at his knee I first learned of the great novels like Charles Dickens *A Tale of Two Cities*, *Oliver Twist* and *Great Expectations* and Mark Twain's *Huckleberry Finn*. Dad was so eloquent in his expression when he read or told us stories he wove a charm around me. He would quote from Shakespeare's sonnets and plays and words took on a magical quality. I can still see him walking around the house, waving his hands in the air, wearing the prissiest of expressions on his face as he recited from *As You Like It*:

All the world's a stage,
And all the men and women merely players.
They have their exits and their entrances;
And one man in his time plays many parts.

As the memory of dad prancing around the room slowly shed a warm light on the icy fear and heaviness in my heart, I realised my father had in his time played many parts. He should've been on the stage; he was *that* good at bringing words and characters to life. But he'd become too busy with his role of husband, father, provider, carer, teacher and accountant to explore other things. I still marvel today at how someone with dad's accountant's brain could be equally great in the literary and language worlds. But I guess that's the complexity of human nature. We are never one thing and, like Shakespeare said, we 'play many parts.'

As dad brought to life characters from books and plays, words from poetry, lyrics and songs I was sucked deeper into the delight of words and storytelling. I was a pre-schooler when I decided I wanted to be an author. English was my favourite subject at school. Words, to me, felt like powerful treasures that could either uplift or deflate.

Under dad's guidance we were taught to mind our p's and q's. We were encouraged from very young to master spelling and to use proper grammar. We were, in fact, encouraged to always work hard; nothing but our best effort was accepted by dad. An average grade was acceptable if we'd tried our best. But we'd feel the sternness of his very long lectures for weeks if we achieved below par due to laziness.

One of my dad's favourite musicals is *My Fair Lady* and a song he played (ad nauseum) was 'Why can't the English?' He'd walk around the lounge room pronouncing the lyrics with the same precise, haughty tone Rex Harrison used and held his right hand with the thumb upwards and firmly resting against the pointy finger it looked like he was pointing both fingers as he waved while enunciating every word. You'd swear he'd been invited to the royal court to entertain the Queen of England.

I spent a lot of time with my dad as a young child badgering him for more stories and poetry. My siblings to this day say I was his favourite. I think we grew close through our love of literature and words. When I look back now, I forced dad into paying attention to me more because I never left him alone. I was curious and hungry for knowledge; always wanted more stories, and I adored him. I think he knew that he was the epitome of wisdom to me.

It was dad who taught me to play chess and I fast became the chess champion in our household. He guided me to check every move, to study the positions of every piece and to ensure my King was protected without being trapped. I thrived on the mental energy of the game and if he hadn't insisted at times that it was bedtime I could easily have played through the night.

Years later while living in LA I was a spectator at an outdoor chess game set up outside of the Starbucks in Ladeira Heights. There was never a shortage of players trying to out manoeuvre each other. These hard-nosed guys sporting various coloured bandanas (signalling the gang they belonged to) would sometimes gather around to watch a chess face-off. Perhaps the gentlemanly tradition of chess travelled through the centuries to envelop even the wayward street thug because I never once saw a fight break out around the game. Chess seemed one non-violent way to get respect from their opposition as well as the onlookers.

As I watched I could see a checkmate move for the player who had a few less pieces left on the board. Before my brain computed I was smack in the middle of 'boys in the hood', I'd made a comment out loud. There was a sudden silence. Was it because a 'mere female' had dared to open her mouth? I'm not sure, but within minutes, I was challenged to a game. Apparently I was to challenge the champion. Amid murmurs and giggles, mostly from the female onlookers, I think all expected the game to be over in two minutes flat.

But what they didn't expect was that their champion was about to play someone who'd been trained by one of the sharpest and, sometimes bordering on the obsessive-compulsive, most precise minds who had trained me very well. It took me a while, but I did eventually enjoy the pleasure of announcing 'check mate.' My friend who was with me at the time told me I was naïve for taking on the gang member; she was sure there'd be some retribution for kicking some gangster butt in a chess game. But I wasn't worried. I saw the admiration and respect in his eyes and I heard the mumbled, 'You're some kinda sister' when I got up to leave.

Besides, some things in the world still command a certain amount of etiquette and respect and chess is one of them. Even if the participants can't always be described as such, the gentleman's rules of play and conduct still apply.

So whether it was language, maths or games dad insisted on best efforts and certainly gave his best when passing on knowledge. He could never be accused of being one of the English who couldn't teach their children how to speak.

Ordinary Man

I'm an ordinary man,
Who desires nothing more than an ordinary chance,
to live exactly as he likes, and do precisely what he wants...
An average man am I, of no eccentric whim,
Who likes to live his life, free of strife,
doing whatever he thinks is best, for him.

('I'm an Ordinary Man' from *My Fair Lady*)

As the range of emotions continued to unravel within me in the twenty-four hours after dad's diagnosis I started to think about the man he really is. He often described himself as ordinary but, every so often, I've thought about his life and seen an ordinary man who does seemingly little things in extraordinary ways.

Now this could be construed as bias — this is, after all, a tribute to my dad. But the tribute means I would not insult him by portraying him as perfect and flawless. Dad's not one who expends a lot of energy worrying about how he'll be perceived. He's king of his castle and none of us have ever been in any doubt about that, including mum. There's a reason he loved the opening verses of 'I'm an ordinary man' from *My Fair Lady*. Dad's always been that man who 'lives exactly as he likes' and does 'precisely what he wants.' And he's never made any apologies for it.

Another reason dad loved the song is, I think, because it elevates men and mocks women. My dad definitely has chauvinistic tendencies. Sometimes he'd make derogatory comments about women just to see our reaction. His eyes would twinkle with glee as he'd quote from the song and when it, sometimes, sparked a debate or reaction from the women in his life, he'd belly laugh to see us riled up. Then, to add salt to our outraged wounds he'd innocently add, 'But I'm a man who has the milk of human kindness by the quart in every vein.' He has been chased about the room or whacked on the head by mum many, many times. His daughters have, on occasion, stomped off in frustration while he laughed so hard his false teeth almost flew from his mouth.

He would take great pleasure in telling me in my teens that I'd some day find a man exactly like him. Of course, I'd adamantly disagree 'Never, ever. That's never going to happen!'

And the first loves I've had have been as far removed from my dad's personality as I could get. Yet, I see now, that those relationships in the end didn't compliment or elevate me as a woman. I'm a wilful, feisty woman who knows exactly what she wants and not all the men I've known have appreciated or even liked that quality in me. I spent a fair chunk of my time trying to play small; trying to avoid putting egotistical noses out of joint. But it always felt like I was short-changing myself.

Now, the man I'm with is a lot like my dad. He's been my best friend for the past five years and is constantly encouraging me to pursue my goals and dreams; has helped me achieve many of them. And he's as responsible, as focused, as intelligent and as warped in his sense of humour as my dad. They're even both Librans. After all the years of trying to figure out what I was looking for in a man, seems I'd have figured it out a lot sooner if I'd looked to my dad. Funny, what we try to run from is often exactly what we need.

Maybe it was the other side, the impatient, bad-tempered, sometimes condescending side of dad that I feared as a child, was what I was running from.

Dad lived by the 'my way or the highway' approach and, once he decided on a way of action, didn't like to be opposed. He and mum would argue over how things should be done and especially how money should be spent. He's always been prudent and hates spending unnecessarily — actually sometimes he's so tight he hates spending even when it's necessary.

A standing family joke is the one about 'five cents' and my dad. Our first sum of pocket money from dad was five cents per week. And he tried to keep that amount going for years. To this day we tease him that 'five cents' is his favourite spending amount. If he says something's too expensive someone will quip, 'What? Was it more than five cents?'

He's headstrong and stubborn with a foul temper (I'd often call him 'Hitler' in my head). Punishment from dad was delivered in one of four ways. He'd withhold our pocket money; tan our bottoms with his slipper; deliver long, drawn out lectures on good or bad behaviour and their consequences or when we were really naughty give us a whipping with the 'proverbial iron rod'. Well, iron cord, really. A black rubber cord from one of mum's old, broken irons was hung on the back of the kitchen door. We feared that cord like you would a snake and would do all we could to avoid the sting of its swish across any part of our body. We hated the ironing cord but at times his long lectures came a close second to the worst punishments of all time. A few times I'd be so fatigued from the lecture as long as Homer's *Iliad* and *Odyssey* combined, I'd wish for the black iron cord instead.

A few days ago, I spoke to dad and on one of his down days since the diagnosis. He was in the 'why me?' frame of mind. It was interesting to hear that he felt like there was an expectation that he would suddenly undergo a massive transformation in his personality; that since he'd been diagnosed with such a grave illness he would become a 'touchy-feely' guy who never got angry anymore. And, while he did understand that anger and stress weren't going to help his healing journey, and he was working on bringing more calm into his life through meditation, he didn't feel he was going to make any major changes in his life. He was, he admitted, a grumpy bugger; had been for most of his life and couldn't see that disappearing in a cloud of enlightenment just because cancer had come knocking.

In trying to come to terms with the disease, he's making changes to improve his spiritual and mental wellbeing, but he's also dealing with feeling anger and confusion that he even has to face this disease. He's always prided himself on his excellent health until now. I'm sure he's disappointed with his body for letting him down. I know I am. I counted on dad's fitness routines to keep him strong well into his eighties or nineties. I always figured he'd be one of those codgers who'd die of natural causes. I never pictured him challenged with a serious illness.

Dad's never had a problem admitting to his shortcomings, even mocking them at times or just choosing not to change them, even if he could. I've always admired his self-awareness and his honesty. He's forthright to the point of bluntness and has no problem in stating his opinions on anything or anyone. Political correctness is not a cloak he wears often, if at all. The people who call him friend are people who admire that honesty and integrity. They never expect him to tip toe around saying what he feels. As a result, dad's not surrounded by loads of fair weather friends. The few who have been in his life have been with him through all seasons and have proven especially loyal through foul weather.

I know dad will listen to and evaluate opinions from friends and experts as he moves forward to confront his biggest battle yet. But I have no doubt he will continue to do whatever 'he thinks is best for him.'

Climb every Mountain

Climb ever mountain, search high and low
Follow every byway, every path you know.
Climb every mountain, ford every stream
Follow every rainbow, till you find your dream.

('Climb every mountain' from *The Sound of Music*)

My earliest memory of going to the movies — probably in primary school — was seeing *The Sound of Music* with my parents. We loved it; saw it probably half a dozen times if memory serves me. The walls of our house were filled with my dad's whistles to the tunes from the musical for months and the song I most associate with dad from that movie, is 'Climb every mountain.'

In so many ways his encouragement of me, to have a go at things, comes from those lyrics. I remember thinking I could, in fact, climb every mountain. I even climbed Table Mountain in Cape Town in a pair of my Sunday best shoes the very first time dad took me on a hiking excursion. I wonder now if it was his warped, bordering on sadistic sense of humour that had him refrain from telling me to wear more sensible shoes like runners. Or if he genuinely didn't notice that I'd left the house with my hiking pack firmly strapped to my back wearing my buckled, white Sunday shoes.

For most kids, the first time for anything means uncontained excitement, restless energy and incessant chanting of 'Are we there yet?' I was no different. Dad noticed I was wearing the 'wrong' shoes only when the cars were parked at Kirstenbosch Gardens at the base of the mountain where the Skeleton Gorge hiking route began. The other impatient hikers in our party were not going to turn back just for a pair of shoes for the newcomer. And I was so keen to get started I convinced him I would be fine. Not that he discouraged me much. He just told me my feet were going to be very sore by the end of the day. But what kid bursting with enthusiasm believes that — especially one itching to place their foot on that first step of a very steep trail. It definitely didn't occur to me there might be a clue in the name of the trail. If I'd thought about 'Skeleton' maybe I'd have understood the implications of danger. Then, I may have lost all courage.

I was amongst the first of our party to begin the climb up the mountain but I didn't remain in the front for long. I soon realised dad wasn't joking about the sore feet. We weren't thirty minutes up the steep track when I started inwardly cursing my pretty white shoes. The square tap-dance style heels on my shoes were not fit to navigate a damp trail along the forest ravine of the gorge. I'd stumbled a few times, but determinedly pushed on. I wasn't about to miss out on my first hike.

Up till then, the adults had been trekking behind the children and teenagers. They slowly overtook me. Dad was amongst the last on the trail, even though he was fit enough to power up the trail with not much effort. But as a responsible man he kept behind when youngsters were along on the hikes.

It didn't take him long to notice I was struggling in my shoes. Before he had a chance to ask if I wanted to turn back I stubbornly let him know I wanted to do the hike. He didn't argue with me, but he never left my side. I can't remember the number of times we had to stop because I stumbled, got tired, had to have a drink or came close to tears. Thankfully, most of Skeleton Gorge trail is densely shaded with thick indigenous trees and forest so it's cool most of the way up. I'm not sure I would've continued if I'd had to deal with the strong African sun beating down on my head.

About half way up the gorge the ladder trail begins. Dad was behind me and encouraged me to keep climbing, keep going up. I must've needed the affirmations; I started chanting 'Up, up, up' all the way up the ladder trail. Near the top of the gorge the trees thin out and from this point I could see the spectacular views over False Bay and the Constantia Valley all the way to the Hottentots Holland Mountains. I was awestruck and momentarily forgot about the discomfort and pain. I could almost have said the pain was worth it — almost.

We still had to scramble over the rocky path near Breakfast Rock though. I tore my eyes from the views across the bay and looked down. That wasn't a smart thing to do because we were on the edge of a cliff drop. Any wrong footing and it would be all too easy to go over. I knew they wouldn't hold over those unpredictable rocks so I took my shoes and my socks off and scrambled the rocks barefoot. By the time we were done, my feet were really hurting. And since we had a lengthy walk ahead to catch up with the others and the path was strewn with brambles and twigs I had to put my socks and shoes back on. Besides I was terrified of snakes and wasn't going to leave my feet exposed to any unfriendly, slithering creatures.

We were the last to reach Maclears Beacon, the highest point of Table Mountain and I had to put up with loads of teasing from the other youngsters. Including their repeating my 'Up, up, up' chant. To this day, when our family recounts my first hiking trip in my white, buckled Sunday shoes, they end with 'Up, up, up' and we fall into fits of laughter.

That first hike with dad up Table Mountain instilled two important things in my life. — First is a deep appreciation and respect for nature — I have found wonder, awe and magic on many a hiking or bushwalking trail. The sounds of mountain springs bubbling over rocks, gentle breezes rustling forest leaves and forest creatures singing, chirping or snapping their wings to communicate are, to this day, the sounds I turn to when my spirit needs rejuvenation or my mind needs respite and a new perspective. I have often brought many troubles and challenges to nature's door and have never left a forest, beach, lake or waterfall empty handed. She has always restored my spirit and often given me an insight I didn't have before I lay my head on her comforting bosom.

The other important thing I gained that day was the first of many instances where I knew I could count on my dad. He never left my side and coached me to the top of that mountain, no matter how painful it was. And he hadn't lied about the sore feet at the end of the day. The blisters I nursed for the days following that hike often saw me in tears. My favourite Sunday shoes were destroyed and I was only too happy to get rid of them. After all, something had to take the blame for my blistered, aching feet.

I was introduced to a method dad consistently applied throughout my life. It is his habit, when asked for advice, to assess a situation only once, provide his opinion and then step back and allow us to make our own decisions. But he's never far away, often lurking in the background ready to help or guide. He will not, however, encourage us to abandon the course of action once the decision has been made. I think he's always had the innate wisdom and belief that we had to learn to climb the mountains in our lives, never give up, because much like that spectacular view over the bay and valleys, the lessons learned are priceless and have stood us in good stead for other challenging experiences along life's trail.

Daddy's Hands

Daddy's hands were soft and kind
When I was cryin'.
Daddy's hands, were hard as steel
When I'd done wrong.
Daddy's hands weren't always gentle
But I've come to understand
There was always love in Daddy's hands.

('Daddy's Hands' — *Holly Dunn*)

It was through the love and nurturing of my dad's hands that my feet healed from the pain and blisters after my first hike up Table Mountain. That wasn't the first time dad made things better with the caring in his hands. Dad was often the one who bathed us at night when we were infants and toddlers. I can't remember him bathing me, but I do remember him bathing my youngest sister. I was seven years old when she was born so my memories of her infant and toddler years are a lot stronger than those of my own.

Dad would often let me help bath her and it was a wonderfully fun routine. He'd soap her hair and let me style it into soapy peaks. Bath time was also singing time. She must've liked that time because she would lie back in the bath gurgling as he'd whistle and sing everything from the Beatles songs, to Frank Sinatra to lyrics from the many musicals he loved. Most of it was off-key, I might add, but I don't think it mattered much to her. She never liked being taken out of the bath and would curl her bottom lip down and scream at the top of her lungs. He'd carry her in the big fluffy towel and lay her down on the bed and then he'd massage her with baby oil. Sometimes he'd let me help massage her back. She would stop crying as soon as the massage routine began. As soon as she was settled and relaxed he'd dress her in her night clothes and lay her in the cot. She'd fall asleep very quickly. If she was a little restless he'd just pat her back for a while and she'd drift off to sleep with her thumb in her mouth and her bum in the air.

Though my memories of dad bathing me are vague, I do remember him washing my hair as a little girl. He would use long, attachable shower pipes to wash our hair, over the bath, every few days. I hated it and would cry the whole time with my eyes tightly shut.

When he'd finally finish rinsing my hair and was squeezing the water from it, I'd open my eyes and say 'Dere, daddy finish.' My siblings tease me about it to this day, especially since I still dislike washing my hair. I much prefer someone else taking care of my hair and I love a good head massage — a treat I came to love through dad who would give my head a quick massage before he combed it after washing. (A favourite pamper these days is my six-weekly visits to the hairdresser to allow someone else to care for my hair.)

Through colds, flus or injuries dad's hands were never far away. He'd rub our chests, back and feet with Vicks Vapour Rub when we were down with a cold or flu. He'd soothe backaches, sports injuries or tight shoulders with Deep Heat or Tiger Balm as we became more physically active through our older years. To this day my sisters and I will often plant our bodies at his feet and beg for a shoulder or back massage when we're stressed or tense. Years later mum, dad and I did a Reiki course together and those who got to be the guinea pig for dad during the practice sessions would compliment him on his healing and nurturing hands.

These traits speak about how complex my dad is. Even as a teen I used to watch him and see such paradoxical traits and be puzzled by them. On the one hand he was stubborn, often angry and aggressive and seemingly emotionless. On the other, there'd be so many moments of tenderness, nurturing and gentleness, that I would often be puzzled by him. But these opposing traits weave through the fabric of his life. They create the mantle of this dear man and he is held together by all the threads of his personality — the harsh course threads and the delicate, dainty ones.

It isn't hard, as I get older, to figure out where some of the harsher traits may have come from. Dad's father was a hard nut to crack. He died when I was very young so I never knew my grandpa. From the stories I've heard, I'm not sure I would've liked knowing him. When my dad was four years old, his mother died. And my grandpa put him and his siblings into an orphanage.

So — through death and through abandonment — dad lost both parents at a young age. Dad had, according to a story mum told us, cried so much when his mum died that his dad threatened to put him in his mother's coffin if he didn't quit. A burning rage rises in me when I think of that; if my grandpa was alive I'd probably want to punch him square in the face for that. And, I especially felt that recently when dad told me he hadn't cried much since being told he had cancer. He wanted to, he said, but somehow couldn't. He'd only cried a bit when he told my daughter, his only grandchild. And it makes sense that crying for dad would never have felt safe, not with a threat like that from his childhood. I wish I could wave a magic wand and put someone in his life who would've comforted him through his childhood grief. I think the source of the man he's become lies in those earlier years.

I've seen, from my own experiences, that intense pain, when not healed, can lead to years of anger and frustration. It can lead to aggression. And it can lead to a desire to compensate or even overcompensate. I suspect dad's softer side was his way of wanting to ensure we felt loved and cared for. What he found difficult to express in words, he communicated through his hands. I don't remember him telling us he loved us very often. And I know he didn't say it much to mum. But when he washed my hair or rubbed me out with balms when I was sick or injured, I always felt his love and caring through his hands.

Years later, when I was broken in mind, body and spirit after splitting with my daughter's father while four months pregnant, the greatest healing came through dad's hands. He'd never approved of that relationship; felt, adamantly, that I deserved better. But I was so headstrong at that time, his disapproval caused the only break my dad and I have ever experienced in our relationship. We didn't speak to each other for a year. It was one of the most painful times in my life. He wouldn't look at me when I visited and would often leave the room when I entered. I can't remember how it was healed, but I was grateful when it was.

When I was thirty, it was my year of crucifixion and glory — truly the worst and best of times. Dad had always stated that once we moved out of home we weren't to come running home again; we were to forge our own way in the world. I'd been away from home for almost eight years by then. But when the relationship with my ex ended, I was pregnant and alone. And I knew I didn't have to ask if I could come back home. The moment my world came crashing down that way, my parents were the first ones to the rescue and though I tried to protest that I'd be alright and would sort something out, dad insisted that I come home for a while. It was through my parents' love and support that I enjoyed a relatively healthy pregnancy. I didn't hear a single 'I told you so' from dad. He simply offered to massage me and give me healing treatments. He helped to heal my broken heart and spirit. I don't think he has any idea how greatly he contributed to mending the shattered pieces of my life, but once again daddy's hands brought comfort like few things could.

I learned something amazing from the paradoxical sides of my dad. As wounded, scarred and flawed as his spirit has been from the age of four, somewhere he has found the ability to still contribute nurturing, caring and love. He might struggle with the emotional words at times, but his hands have always been able to convey what his lips weren't able to. And I've always felt the 'love in daddy's hands.'

Ebony and Ivory

Ebony and ivory
live together in perfect harmony.
Side by side on my piano keyboard,
or lord, why don't we?

('Ebony and Ivory' — *Paul McCartney and Stevie Wonder*)

The first time I saw anxiety on my father's face and realised he wasn't invincible was when I was seven. It was a hot summer's day and we'd gone to Gordon's Bay beach, in South Africa, with family friends. My siblings and I were building sandcastles on the shore while the grown-ups rested in the shade of a tree. I was having a great deal of fun, building the biggest sandcastle I could and was obviously far too young to notice that the beach was largely abandoned.

That was until my view was obstructed by black shoes and navy trousers. And harsh, angry tones yelled in Afrikaans, 'Wat doen julle hier? (What are you doing here?)' The first face I looked for was my dad's. The clenching of his jaw, his body rigid and the anger, controlled but pure, on his face frightened me. I wanted to cry, but knew, in that moment, I shouldn't; nothing felt safe — not even crying. I did not move.

Here stood two police officers pointing to a sign on the beach. Within moments the grown-ups hurriedly gathered our picnic blanket and belongings and summoned us to go. Though none of the children wanted to leave, we knew not to protest or question our parents. It was probably one of the few times we sprang to obedience when told to 'come.' As our cars drove off the beach parking lot, I turned to look back at the sign the police officers had pointed to. It read 'NET

BLANKES' on the left side of the sign with its English translation of 'WHITES ONLY' on the right. It was the first time I noticed my skin wasn't chocolate anymore. Something felt wrong with it — like it was tarnished, tainted and dirty. It had lost its chocolate delight.

I could tell that leaving that beach was not what my dad had wanted to do. I sensed he had wanted to punch those policemen. I wondered why he didn't. I was too young to know that leaving, however humiliating, was the safest course of action at that time, especially for us children.

Today, as I raise my daughter in Melbourne, Australia, I think about what it must've felt like for my parents to raise children in a country infested with apartheid; a country scourged with racial segregation and bigotry. How would they have struggled to build self-esteem in children of colour in a country where laws, signs and attitudes scream 'inferior' and 'not welcome' to anyone not white skinned.

Even in Australia, I sometimes find it challenging keeping my daughter's belief in herself elevated since she's different looking to the average blonde, blue-eyed child in our neighbourhood. And we live in one of the most cosmopolitan cities in the world.

The constitutional laws of Australia forbid such bigotry, but, growing up in a country like South Africa in the 60s, 70s and 80s I was always aware that the apartheid system ensured there were limits on my potential to achieve in that country. Most people of colour who gained any kind of accolades in their respective fields had to leave South Africa to do so. Yet, as the hold of apartheid began to slowly loosen in the early 80's, the threats and incidence of violence grew. It came from unexpected quarters; from the unemployed, from angry youth whose respect for life and property had been so severely tested under apartheid that violence seemed a viable option. I know that my parents were increasingly alarmed by it and worried constantly for our safety.

After that first encounter with such overt racism that day on the beach, at seven I badgered my dad. I wanted answers for why such bad behaviour was allowed. He was never able to explain it in a way that satisfied my desire to understand. Perhaps he didn't understand it either. He would rage when he experienced prejudice; also when he saw or heard of others who were discriminated against or, even abused, because of their skin colour. In the safety of our home, he would scream curses — usually about white people — as he stomped about and waved his arms raging against every white man, their ancestors, children and animals. And then, every day, he'd have to return to his work— a place owned and run by white men and women. When I was younger, I'd wonder how he behaved at work. I figured he hadn't been calling his employers names or he'd probably be fired. It was only in my early teens when I got my first job through dad, helping out with filing and other office duties at his workplace that I got to see him in action around white people. He was the company's accountant and office administrator; in some ways, understood the company and its people better than the owners did. And he always carried himself with pride. His intelligence and hard work shone through.

Dad commanded respect from everyone. Not only is he able to learn things very quickly, he is also a gifted teacher; able to teach what he knows effectively to people at different levels of comprehension. I'd see him sit down with the company's executives and explain the figures, talk about best practices for growing the company as they all sat in the comfort of air-conditioned meeting rooms. Hours later I'd see him out in the dusty quarry yards talking to the labourers and, no doubt, teaching them things. The black labourers often referred to my dad as 'baas' even though they knew he wasn't the owner of the company.

In much of South Africa, in those days, most of the black labourers had to leave their families behind in rural areas and go to the big cities to find work. They tended to live in cramped and sub-standard housing in 'townships' and, more often than not, worked long and hard for very little money. They didn't mingle easily with races outside of their own.

The basis of apartheid, the grounds on which the then Afrikaaner government ruled the peoples of South Africa, was a division by race. Whites were, automatically, top of the pile. Blacks were declared the lowest and considered and treated worse than most white people's pets. In the middle, then, came those classified as 'coloured' — a term applied to anyone of mixed race. My birth certificate states I am officially 'Cape Coloured' and this deliberate dividing of races worked exceptionally well for white people. But it left its scars on the rest of us. When words or attitudes are repeated over and over; be it overtly or subliminally; they are eventually absorbed into the subconscious mind and it is from this place that we often create our world. Black and coloured people were constantly reminded of how inferior they were as a race. After a while they would either act and behave in ways that perpetuated this thinking (being submissive and bowing down to white people) or they would try desperately to elevate their status and, if they succeeded, lord it over those they thought were beneath them.

Sometimes 'coloured' folk were as intolerant of black people as whites were. Racial bigotry was a festering sore that bred fear in people and that in turn led to ugly behaviour across all races, even amongst our own kind. People would often try to elevate their 'colour' status by the shades of skin colour. Bizarre, but understandable. Many fair skinned coloureds who could pass for white certainly did everything they could to enjoy the privileges reserved for white South Africans. And they weren't above selling out their own people or the blacks for those treasures. Blacks often mistrusted coloureds as much as they did the whites.

This made it somewhat surprising to witness the respect the black labourers had for my dad and how easily they let him into their circles. One day, on lunch break at work, I walked around the quarry and ran into a few of the labourers sitting on the side of the quarry eating their lunch. 'Hey, you baas Nick's daughter?' asked one man. When I nodded he invited me to sit with them. I was nervous and didn't know what to do. I'd heard the stories of blacks hating whites, but also disliking coloureds intensely. I'd also heard some of the older coloured people in our neighbourhood talk about blacks in unflattering ways. They'd say things like 'you can't trust a darkie or a kaffir' or 'those blacks always want something from you — a handout.' At the time I was too young to see that this fearful behaviour was part of the ramifications of a racially segregated society, so as a youngster I kept to my coloured community and was as suspicious of blacks as I was of whites.

So that day I was torn between curiosity and suspicion. Curiosity won and I walked over cautiously and sat on a boulder next to him. He offered me some of his buttermilk. I wasn't a lover of milk and told him so. Buttermilk, he promised, was different and I'd like it. I took a swig. It tasted like liquid yoghurt. The delight on my face must've shown. The next thing he did was pour half his buttermilk into a tin cup and offer it to me. And then Gageele, introduced himself and proceeded to tell me what a good man my dad was. His charcoal face broke into a huge smile and he had sparkling white teeth (was it all the buttermilk?). He dipped this grainy, almost black bread into his buttermilk and ate that meal as though it'd been specially prepared by the most accomplished chefs. In between slopping up his bread and buttermilk, he shared anecdotes of how my dad helped the black workers. Whether it was talking to the 'big baas' on their behalf or explaining things to them in a way they understood — dad was always trying to make sure the labourers got a fair and honest deal in their working life. To this day whenever I see buttermilk in the stores I think of that first time I drank it with Gageele and I see the brightest white teeth flashing the biggest smile as he spoke about 'baas Nick.'

The owners of the company approached dad with the kind of respect I never expected to see from white men. I'd see them approach him with caution, never wanting to intrude on his time. Dad was so focused and dedicated to the tasks at hand in his every day working life, he didn't pause for unnecessary chit-chat with anyone, including his bosses. It seemed they knew and valued the fact that dad was a dedicated worker who got the job and so much more done. They knew their company was thriving largely because of how dad ran the day-to-day operations and how he got the best out of their labourers.

When it came to socialising, our circles were confined to our own coloured community. We didn't mingle much with whites or indeed blacks. We did however get to know some through our working life. As angry as my dad got behind closed doors about injustice, racism and bigotry in South Africa he took the 'educate them one person at a time' approach when dealing with whites. He guided and influenced his bosses in subtle ways to fair, honest and humane dealings with all the workers in the company regardless of skin colour. He always gave his best and then some and stood tall and proud. I know he never 'played the victim card' and was comfortable in his own skin. And that, I believe, is how he commanded such respect wherever he worked.

Dad could've chosen to become a political activist and joined the many causes in the fight for freedom for the oppressed people in South Africa. But he used his talents as a teacher, rather — as someone who influenced and educated people in a more personal way. Education and knowledge was dad's path to freedom. Illiteracy was a large problem among blacks in South Africa at that time and dad volunteered to teach reading and writing in the black townships, working with nuns and other lay people. Dad believed in the ripple effect of education — his help for just one person might mean they in turn helped another in their community, and before long an entire community is uplifted from the clutches of illiteracy and helplessness.

I learned valuable lessons from dad in so many ways but, in this realm, it was about how to deal with ugliness of behaviour. I learned that retaliation and violent reactions only lead to more ugliness. Sometimes the best way to change something is to adopt Gandhi's sage advice and 'become the change you wish to see in the world.' In his own way dad tried to help ebony and ivory live side by side even when the laws of the land espoused the opposite.

Redemption Song

Emancipate yourselves from mental slavery
None but ourselves can free our mind

('Redemption Song' — *Bob Marley*)

Even while dad tried to advocate integration amongst black and white I also saw him trying daily to rise above the oppressive environment of apartheid. Yet for all his efforts neither he nor his children could fully escape the emotional and mental scars of such overt bigotry, hatred and violence.

From my first shock of realising we were to be treated differently on that summer's day at the beach, I struggled to understand that kind of behaviour. I wondered what God had made the rules that allowed one race dominance over another. As a young child I'd often talk to God and ask him why this was happening in my country and why he wasn't doing anything about it. I started writing stories and poetry. But they weren't fairytales; they were often dark and gloomy and almost always involved an escape of sorts — that's where the fantasy was quite elaborate. I used to wish I could escape my skin colour. Once I learned my skin wasn't chocolate anymore, I lost the carefree feelings of early childhood. I became an adult in a girl's body long before my time.

Sometimes I mourn the loss of that innocence, that freedom. As I watched my daughter as a little girl in her childhood play; listening to her made-up tales of mermaids, fairies and fantastical creatures, I loved witnessing the magical moments of awe and wonder woven through her playtime. I often wonder what it would've felt like to experience that as a child. Instead my young girl's thoughts were plagued with unanswered questions. I was an intense child who grew into a brooding teenager and a very serious young adult.

From when I was a teenager, I was aware of my dark skin and I wasn't comfortable being in it. No matter how many questions I asked — of God, of my dad, of my teachers — nobody gave me any satisfying answers. As the years went by and more incidents of prejudice and maltreatment followed, my confusion turned to hurt, anger and fear. Perhaps the worst part of growing up in South Africa, at that time, with the intensely oppressive policy that apartheid was, was feeling trapped — like there was no other way.

I think the greatest tragedy of this experience is realising that even though we didn't feel right, often we did little, or even nothing to change it. Accepting this way of life like a force that couldn't be countered scarred us as a race more, I think, than the outright acts of hatred and bigotry inflicted upon us. For a long time black people in South Africa endured the bitter wounds of oppression and violence. Our apathy and acceptance of a vile and sick situation; our collective unconscious of silent agreement, the tacit acceptance and failure to question and to act, meant we were trapped. Trapped and feeling helpless.

My dad would often try to encourage us. 'You are as good as anyone', he'd say. But the bizarre thing was that it never left me feeling encouraged. It was only years later when reading Dr Martin Luther King Jr's autobiography, that I understood why. In the book, Luther King Jr states that the mere use of the phrase 'you are as good as anyone' speaks of the injustice that makes its use necessary. As a youngster, my reaction to that phrase was often a simple 'bullshit!' Because the laws of the land clearly stated that we weren't as good as anyone.

As the chains of apartheid tightened and its effects bound my mind and everyday life, I began to hunger for my freedom. At first, the simple freedoms. I longed to be able to go into any cinema, sit in any train carriage or go to any school. I started dreaming of going to another place — anywhere, but South

Africa. America with its slogan 'the land of the free and home of the brave' became a desired destination.

But, wishing to be somewhere else, yet knowing there wasn't a way out, wasn't the only burden I carried as a teenager. I had enough self awareness to feel hostage in a sense, to an ominous cloud of inferiority. In my later years I could grasp Eleanor Roosevelt's words *'no one can make you feel inferior without your consent'* — but as a child and teen I couldn't. So I struggled with the crushed feelings I experienced every time I bore the brunt of a dismissal, a sour look, a foul word; every time I saw others having to endure them. I allowed the fears and hatred from others to seep into my young mind. I took on the idea that there was something ugly and unworthy about me and the colour of my skin.

One day, in my teenage years, I was roughly shoved off a train by an uncompromising white conductor because, out of desperation to catch the train, more than anything, I'd dared to jump into the 'whites only' carriage. Not that he understood that. My connecting bus for school had been late so I was running to get the train and not be late for school. I don't know what I feared more — the nuns reprimand for being late or being caught in the 'wrong' carriage.

The train had barely pulled out of the station when I was caught by the conductor. He marched me roughly through the carriage and forced me off the train at the next stop. I cried with the humiliation and the anger of it. I scanned the carriage looking for just one sympathetic face; there were none. When I eventually got to school, I was so angry at what had happened that I offered no explanation for my tardiness and simply stared defiantly at the school principal when she asked why I was late. I forced back hot tears stinging the back of my eyes as she called me 'rebellious' and 'troublesome' and handed me a detention slip.

I didn't immediately share this incident with my dad or anyone else in my family. Though dad and I had always talked easily to each other about most things, somehow I couldn't bring myself to burden him with it. And I didn't want him to see the deep pain and anger building within me.

In the meantime darkness crept deeper and deeper into my soul. One day, when I was sixteen, I changed very dramatically. I collapsed. Those around me thought I was distressed because I was having trouble with a girl at school. And, while it may have been a contributing factor or perhaps the straw that broke the camel's back, I knew my soul had been hurting long before that. What I understand now is that those years of suppressed anger, hatred and pain of what I witnessed and what I experienced culminated in a deep, dark depression.

I remember feeling sad all the time for months before it all finally came crashing. But I hid it well. I'd always been the one whose nose was buried in books or was curled up in a corner writing poetry and stories, so there was no unusual behaviour to warn my parents of what was really going on. I was walking down the school corridor to English class one day and my legs gave way under me. I was shaking and couldn't make sense of anything around me. I vaguely remember mum and dad taking me home from school. After that, it was as though I lived in a black cloud. I didn't return to school for some time. I don't remember doing much; I do remember sitting in my bedroom staring out of the window. My memories of that time are clouded; fuzzy snippets of mum bringing me food and dad trying to talk to me with little or no response from me. I was in a dark abyss and there was no feeling — no joy, no happiness, no love, no hate, no anger, no hurt — just nothing.

One of the things that stands out the most was that my world had no colours. I would look out the window and see shapes — of plants, trees, the garden — but no colours. Everything merged in a colourless lump. Nothing was clearly defined. And I was in the abyss, shutting out everyone. Not even my beloved father could get in. It was the one time in my life I danced alone — almost.

Somewhere, in the darkness of my depression, I could sense something. It came and went but it felt light and comforting. I can't say for sure what it was, but I decided it must've been a touch of divinity. I can only describe it as 'angelic'. It was nothing I could see or touch, only feel. And every time it arrived a deep peace and lightness would surround me.

Then, one day, that light pulled me out of the dark cloud. And I emerged from my bedroom and I resumed my life unable to explain where I'd been all those weeks or how I had returned to my life. It would be many years before I remembered that light and realised I was protected — even through that time. The realisation that I wasn't alone, even through a time when I couldn't identify myself in the world anymore, has been a source of great comfort to me since. No matter how challenging life has become for me, I've always known that there is light even in the darkest moments.

Surrendering to the dark depression in my own mind and knowing that my soul had been shattered by the sad feelings of inferiority was also the start of my mental emancipation.

I emerged from the abyss stronger and determined to be part of the solution in South Africa and before long was one of the 'troublemakers' leading awareness campaigns at my high school. We — the head prefect and some of my other fellow prefects — became involved in freedom campaigns. My conversations with dad went from literary discussions on Shakespeare, Dickens and Joyce to political discussions about Mandela, Kathrada and Biko. He warned me, naturally, to be aware of the dangers that being politically active might bring. But he also encouraged me to truly understand and be well informed; to make sure education was a primary weapon in my political fight. I should not be following any course blindly, driven only by volatile emotions. Blind passion for anything or anyone, he felt, was dangerous. I agreed with him (to a point) but, as a teenager, I also believed I was invincible. That was until I began to see for myself what lack of education, fuelled by blind passion could lead to.

As the boil of oppression reached bursting point and black people began rallying more and more for their civil rights; as political rallies, picketing, burning tyres in protest became familiar signs of the changing tides, so did police brutality.

Violence escalated. And it seemed we were making strides to free us from the oppressive hand of apartheid. But often it was not towards peace and harmonious integration. I started to see that peaceful change cannot be achieved by violent means and hatred. Many of the victims of political violence and police brutality were innocent people caught in the crossfire of blind hatred and retaliation. And I began to understand the truth in Gandhi's words 'What difference does it make to the dead, the orphans and the homeless, whether the mad destruction is wrought under the name of totalitarianism or the holy name of liberty or democracy?'

There again, I saw the wisdom in my dad's approach of educating and uplifting people through knowledge, rather than inciting them with anger, vengeance and retaliation. There's little or no longevity in gaining anything through violent means or fear. The only structures that survive over time are those built on love, harmony and peace. And we can only move towards love, harmony and peace when we free ourselves from fear and hatred of others and of ourselves. It is our own inner self loathing and negative self talk that enslave us so much more than any external hatred could ever do.

It would take many more years before I freed myself from such powerful mental shackles that branded me inferior. But I had the help of mentors — like my dad, and, a particularly inspiring German teacher who saw me so much bigger than I saw myself. There have been many routes to personal development but it would be years later, in another land, many miles away from my beloved Africa that my soul would find sufficient peace to sing its 'redemption songs.'

Food glorious food

Food glorious food
We're anxious to try it
Three banquets a day
Our favourite diet
Just picture a great big steak
fried, roasted or chewed
For food, marvellous food,
wonderful food, magical food
fabulous food, beautiful food
GLORIOUS FOOD

('Food, glorious food' — from *Oliver*)

Food is the centrepiece around which everything occurs in my family, community and culture. And dad is the patron of food in our circle. Sometimes there's such an abundance of food at our celebrations that there'd be enough to feed a tiny village even after all guests have had seconds and thirds.

Our family table often groaned under the weight of curry dishes, mum's macaroni and cheese (a better one you won't find anywhere), colourful sautéed vegetables, salads, meats, seafood and, usually, more than one dessert. It was a place where family stories were told; and few tales top the one my dad told of his days in the orphanage. Even my daughter now asks grandpa about those days and I notice she wears the same wide-eyed expression I did as a girl soaking up the life and humour of my dad's orphanage tales.

In his young days, poverty hung like a heavy curtain around my dad's family home. After his mother died and he and his siblings were hastily dumped into an orphanage by their father, any chance of tasting the life of a young prince slipped away before he'd learned the word 'royal.'

Dad's passion for food probably began all those years ago, when food was either scarce or boring. Dad tells of thick stews mostly made of peas and thick vinegary gravy plonked onto their plates by the nuns — definitely not something to prompt any of the children asking, as per Oliver's rendition 'Please sir, may I have some more?'

Once a week they'd get a piece of meat in the stew, the size of a grown man's thumb. They'd savour it; try every trick to get an extra piece or someone else's. There'd be bartering, coercing and oftentimes downright theft just to enjoy the chewy texture of another measly portion. Worse than the tiny morsels, though, would be when the nuns removed the tiny portions of meat from the stew before serving leaving just the teasing flavour of meat and, presumably, saving the pieces to reuse for another stew.

But the nun's could bake bread, 'like it was nobody's business', said dad. His favourite smell in the orphanage was that of freshly baked bread. He especially loved the crusty ends of the loaf or, as we call it in Afrikaans, the 'korsie'. He and his friends would sneak into the kitchen and shove pieces of bread down the front of their shirts, then beat a hasty retreat to the nearest hiding spot where they would gobble it down to the tiniest korsie crumb. The greasy stains of butter on their shirts would give them away but, most times, the taste and smell of the warm, moist, freshly-baked bread was worth any punishment they might receive. And he reckoned the nuns expected to find missing bread and young boys with greasy stained shirts in close proximity of the kitchen. Freshly baked bread with a healthy spread of butter and jam is still amongst dad's favourite snacks. And he will fight you tooth and nail for the 'korsie.' Much to mum's frustration, he still makes a mess, with buttered crumbs on his shirt, tracksuit or the couch. The pure delight on his face as he slurps his bread dipped in tea or coffee is like one who gets a covert thrill from doing something forbidden. I'm sure somewhere in his sub-conscious mind, his young self is savouring that stolen bit of bread.

Dad's orphanage tales are rich with the sense of camaraderie that existed with his siblings and his friends. The bonds are strong between these children who had almost nothing, but were never short of entertainment. Boredom was not part of their vocabulary, finding their entertainment in each other and in their invented games from the playgrounds and dorms of the orphanage. The maze of passages they dug in the sandy playground and the underground games they invented no doubt gave birth to some fine young engineers. Dad's only lament is that they could never quite dig a tunnel big enough or long enough from which to escape. Somehow when they got near the fenced perimeters of the orphanage grounds, they always hit concrete blocks or sewage pipes.

Dad and his gang of mischief makers also, he remembers, turned seemingly heavy chores into something fun. The young boys had turns in polishing the marble floor in the church — apparently an arduous task. There was quite a knack to applying a thick beeswax polish in order to keep those floors sparkling like jewels. The trick lay in buffing the floors at a rapid speed — and not allowing the wax time to cake unevenly on the floor. So, inventive and looking for entertainment, dad and his friends tied their cleaning cloths around their feet and skated up and down the floor. For the larger floor surfaces, they would seat one or two of the boys on 'carpets' of bigger towels or cloths and push them over the floor. They got a kick out of using bums and feet to buff the church floor to a mirror shine; it wouldn't be any fun if they hadn't included some kind of mischief. As they neared the end of their task, they would often drag the seated boys around and then, let go suddenly, causing them to fly into church benches or walls while the rest howled with laughter. But, ever fair, they made sure they each got their turn at being flung around the church.

One of the most amusing and touching stories from that time is the story of dad's grey feet. Dad didn't have any shoes as a young boy and would run around barefoot. Before long, the coarse, dark grey sand of the orphanage playground would cake on his feet and leave a coating of mud-like plaster. He wore these 'permanent grey' shoes all the time and, though he may have been teased about the 'grey feet', dad would laugh when he told the story, always ending with his favourite part. This was where his sisters would sit him down every few weeks and use a stone to scrub the grey off his feet. He was being pampered with an orphanage version of a pedicure and exfoliating scrub.

In his first years at the orphanage my dad was the youngest child and was often spoilt by the nuns and some of the older children. Years later when, as an adult, he worked with the nuns in the black townships, he often came home with sweet treats (like coconut ice or macaroons) given to him by the nuns who'd taught him as a boy in the orphanage. He loved to think he still had the charm of his younger years. It's interesting that anything to do with food is still considered the best of treats by dad.

The years apart from his children hadn't changed my grandpa much and when dad and his siblings finally left the orphanage, they only stayed with their father for a short time before moving out and setting up house together in a one-bedroom place.

They spent their teen and young adult years taking care of each other. Dad was the youngest and still in high school when they moved. His role in the household was to cook dinner and have it ready for his working siblings. A sorry tale, one of dad's worst memories he says, was of the time he spoiled the evening meal with a bar of soap. He'd cooked a hot pot of sorts and when he went to stir it, had unknowingly placed the lid over a bar of Sunlight soap (a heavy-duty household cleaning soap). The bar had stuck to the inside of the lid and, by the time the casserole had simmered through, had completely melted into the evening meal. The gag reaction from his siblings was nothing compared to the anger they unleashed on him or the disappointment he felt at having wasted a pot of food. And that distress at waste has not changed in all these years. Dad would sooner eat the same leftovers for days on end than see food go to waste. There's no way he's ever going to abuse his 'glorious food' — not in this lifetime anyway.

That's what friends are for

Keep smilin', keep shinin'
Knowin' you can always count on me, for sure
That's what friends are for
For good times and bad times
I'll be on your side forever more
That's what friends are for

('That's what friends are for' — *Dionne Warwick*)

When it comes to friendships or at least numbers and friends, mum's the one in the household who's led the way. She is mother earth. And people have always gravitated towards her — plus she can cook up a storm at the drop of a hat. And she's been known to almost force-feed folk who walk through her door. You don't leave my mum's kitchen hungry.

Dad has never been surrounded by many friends; probably due to his aloof demeanour and the fact he doesn't suffer fools easily. He has no problem letting someone know they're a fool if the situation or behaviour warrants it. His razor sharp tongue, when crossed and his wit and intelligence, means he can spit sarcasm like a cobra ready to strike. Naturally, people have a tendency to be wary of him and his grumpy, sometimes angry temperament.

But there have always been the few who have looked beyond this protective mantle and taken the trouble to know the whole man. Those who did have remained lifelong friends for they have found dad to be a fiercely loyal, truthful and helpful friend.

One of the boys dad grew up with in the orphanage was mum and dad's best man at their wedding. They'd been through the best and worst and, in their early adult life, exchanged boyish games for bushwalks, mountain hikes, way too much alcohol and skirt chasing. They never abandoned their friendship or the memories that built it.

I've learned a lot about true friendship through witnessing my dad's friendships. Dad's not one to waste time on mindless chatter or frivolity. His conversations, debates and observations with his friends were focused on current affairs, family, children, community, politics, learning and his work. He loved debate (he should've been a lawyer) and never let his emotions get in the way of the facts so he'd debate and rationalise until he won folk over with pure logic — could out argue most people. Two close friends from South Africa remained in his life because they could rise to his challenges, they spoke as frankly as he did and they viewed life with the same warped humour he did.

Both men were, incidentally, reformed alcoholics. Dad had not become one, but had, he said, been a pretty heavy drinker in his teen and young adult years. I suppose with no parents to guide his choices and siblings who were too busy working, he was left to his own devices. He started smoking at a very young age and was consuming alcohol in his mid-teens. Mum always says her mother did not want her to date dad, let alone marry him, because he drank too much. The time he was supposed to spend wooing her, he spent in intoxicated sleep. Mum had grown up with an alcoholic father so her mother was worried she was doomed to the same sorry fate with dad.

But just when you think you've got dad pegged, he'll surprise you. On mum's twenty-first birthday he gave up alcohol. For good. Though he was the barman at her birthday party, ensuring everyone's glass remained merrily filled, he decided he was done with alcohol and hasn't touched liquor since. His only taste of alcohol since that day comes in the small amounts added to Christmas trifles, puddings and cakes.

Though in my teen years, I was surprised to see dad become so close to men who battled the booze, now I understand how his empathy showed through; how the bond was formed. Dad made no judgements. He was always more focused on their recovery and sobriety, rather than the times they fell off the wagon. And the stories they told — oh the stories.

I'd want to sit around in their company because of the way they shared the stories of the alcohol-induced escapades and fumbles. I marvelled at how easily they laughed at themselves and how open and honest they were in sharing everything. From slumping against girls in the middle of slow dances to falling out of buses and falling into bushes, the stories were vibrant with humour and raw with truth. There was no censoring and the gritty truth of their fallibility and struggles endeared them to dad, mum and us children. And our family home was never short of laughter. Anything that brought an extra dose of laughter was always welcome in our home, even if it was the drunken tales of dad's closest buddies.

Years later I was taking a break from my IT career, travelling through California. I was on a visit to the Rochester House and grew interested in the man who once owned it. It had been the sprawling mansion of the late Eddie Anderson, one of the first African-American actors, who won fame playing Rochester, the valet to Jack Benny's character on *The Jack Benny Show* which ran for many years as a radio and television series. Throughout his stellar career in Hollywood when roles for African-American actors were as rare as pink diamonds, he always remembered the challenges he'd faced to attain his dreams and made philanthropy and humanitarian works a priority in his life. One of his last philanthropic gestures was to bequeath his sprawling residence to house 'at risk' homeless substance abusers. His son, Edmund Jr, founded and opened the Rochester House and to this day continues the legacy of his father by providing support and transition programs for people who have battled with mind-altering substances and consequently lost homes, family and friends. When I heard the story behind the

Rochester House it struck a chord with me. Eddie Anderson reminded me a lot of my dad. His will to overcome his challenges and desire to help others touched me. I saw snippets of my dad's life when I listened to his son, Edmund Jr speak of his father's legacy. I was interested and felt drawn to get involved in some of the support programs the Rochester House offered. Before I knew it, I was in conversation with him and within two weeks had started working there as an office administrator.

I'd often chat with the residents in the garden near the swimming pool — some very rough looking, wearing years of substance abuse. They couldn't figure out how a young woman, who'd never touched alcohol or any drugs could empathise so much with their stories. But my journey of empathy with other people's personal struggles had begun years before in the company of dad and his friends. I've always been drawn to the 'real' stuff people share rather than the masks many people wear even though they rarely hide the truth.

I learned about acceptance through dad's friendships. But I also learned about bringing humour to any situation. This healthiest of ingredients has a way of leaving one with a feeling that however bad things may have been, something of value was gained.

Dad's example of acceptance encouraged us in our own friendships. Our home was a sanctuary to many a troubled soul; many came from broken or abusive homes and they spent more of their time in my family's home than their own. I often got teased at school about befriending the troubled, lonely or left-out girls — the strays. Like dad, I was never one to follow the popular crew or adopt the ideas and thoughts of most cliques. But it didn't matter who we brought home — as long as they minded their manners and showed respect, they were always welcome and made to feel like part of the family. An extra setting at the table was never too much trouble.

I don't remember a lot of quiet in our home while growing up nor do I remember extended periods of time with just the seven members of our immediate family. Someone's friend was always stopping over — for a yarn over a quick cup of tea or a lengthy counselling session or, importantly, quiet sanctuary for a broken heart or troubled soul. Often our dining room became a games parlour housing card or board games that lasted for hours. Since none in our family or circle of friends ever gave up easily when it came to out gaming each other, there was more than one occasion when pumpkin time had long passed before anyone turned in for bed.

And at the helm of all the laughter, tears, challenges and fun we shared with friends sat my dad who could always be counted on through good and bad times — always knowing 'that's what friends are for.'

The Prayer

I pray you'll be our eyes, and watch us where we go.
And help us to be wise in times when we don't know
Let this be our prayer, when we lose our way
Lead us to the place, guide us with your grace
To a place where we'll be safe.

('The Prayer' — *Celine Dion and Andrea Bocelli*)

'Cardie' (shortened from Cardinal) was one of dad's nicknames in his early twenties. He was very involved in the Roman Catholic Church and, for a time, attended mass daily. He also sang in the church choir and read from the scriptures at mass. I suppose it was a natural progression from being raised in a Catholic orphanage; the same nuns who spoiled him with treats in his childhood would most likely have impressed on him how important it was to be a good Catholic boy. The name 'Cardie' had been bestowed on dad by his brother-in-law, as a reference to his piousness and his daily walk through the neighbourhood with his bible under his arm on his way to daily mass.

My earliest memories of religion and churches, was walking through our neighbourhood with mum and dad to St Theresa's Catholic Church, the closest one to our home. Every time we went, we got the same stern lecture from our parents to behave and sit quietly in the pews. God forbid we didn't heed the words and mum would either lean over and pinch us or give us the look that meant we were in big trouble. Dad was usually so caught up in the service, rituals and ceremonies that he rarely noticed what we kids were up to. But mum had the bionic eyes and ears. Still, it was dad's long-winded lectures and whippings we feared. So most times we'd sit there bored to tears not daring to glance sideways at each other.

As we grew older we were encouraged by dad to participate in church activities. My two brothers became altar boys, got to swing the incense holder, carry the wine chalices and, at Easter, carry the tall cross around the church as the priest performed the stations-of-the-cross ceremony. That was one of the times I wished I was a boy; they got to do all the fun things. Well, at least they didn't have to sit through service with their hands in their lap wondering how long the priest's sermon was going to last.

St Theresa's Catholic Primary School, next door to the church, was where we went to school. The principal, a nun who'd taught dad briefly in the orphanage, expected more from the Alexander children because of their long association. I had to read at the weekly Wednesday mass most weeks and joined the school choir. But in my last year of primary school, I started rebelling against the principal and the expectations she had of me.

One Wednesday, I and a friend who was also a regular reader, refused to read at mass. It wasn't just to be rebellious or that we were sick of reading. It was also our attempt to stay popular — there'd been complaints and comments to our face and behind our backs from the other kids in our class about not getting a chance to read.

But trying to get that stubborn nun to understand why we were refusing was like undertaking a campaign for women to become priests in the Catholic Church — it was never going to happen. We stood our ground though and refused to leave the school playground to attend the Wednesday mass. We were promptly suspended from school and sent home. Mum wasn't happy to see me come through the door before lunchtime and I know she was embarrassed that I'd dare to challenge the principal that way. I spent the rest of the day confined in the bedroom, haunted by the words 'wait till your dad gets home tonight.' I dreaded the lecture which would surely come and felt certain the iron cord behind the kitchen door was going to be used too.

To my surprise, dad allowed me to explain why I'd refused to read at church and when he realised the other kids at school weren't getting a turn he said he'd talk to the principal. I'm not sure what words were exchanged between them, but I was back in school within two days.

And the next week two other children were given a turn at reading. By the time we finished primary school, all the students in our class and the other grade six class had had a turn. Was it the charm he'd used on the nuns as a boy under their tutelage that worked yet again with the school principal or something else? I suspected it had more to do with his sense of fairness. As stern and as strict as he was as a parent, dad always had a strong sense of fairness; always weighing all sides of any case before deciding on any action. And he would always put up a strong fight to ensure fairness was achieved in any situation.

My rebellion at church, school and related activities didn't stop with that first one against the weekly reading. It was in fact the beginning of my rebellion. I managed to get through my confirmation as a teenager, but just barely. I started questioning a lot of the church doctrine in confirmation classes and was kicked out of Sunday school on more than one occasion. Somewhere in my spirit I wasn't comfortable. Perhaps it was with the fear-based teachings which stated punishment for all sinners who didn't follow the rule.

Yet, despite my rebellion against some Catholic doctrine, I always maintained a very close and spiritual relationship with God. I talked to God all the time about everything. It was a casual affair though — no pious conversation. In fact some 'prayers' often involved curse words when something challenging was going on in my life or the lives of loved ones.

These days I talk to angels; they represent the link, the perfect balance of earthly and heavenly energy. They don't feel as far away as God sometimes felt to me, yet I feel they are his messengers and can translate my messages, requests and prayers more clearly to his divine ear than I sometimes can. It's what works for me.

I was the first one in our family to stop going to church. That was always a given considering my rebellion. It did surprise me when mum and dad stopped going to Sunday mass a few years after we migrated to Australia. Could it be that church was less important? That it had been one of their pillars in life while living through the harsh backdrop of apartheid in South Africa. It's not unusual for people to cling to religion when there's fear or huge challenges. I think it's far more empowering to choose religion or any spiritual practice simply because it instils a sense of peace or enhances the good we already feel inside. I don't believe God or his angels ever meant us to feel anything other than love and peace when we're communing with them.

I've noticed a sense of peace and contentment come over dad when he's pottering around in his garden, out riding his bike and particularly when he's out in nature — either on a hike or walking along beach promenades or tracks. I think he finds it easier to connect to God and to his own spirit when he's out amongst the marvels of nature which we often refer to as God's art.

Since dad was diagnosed with cancer, he's started daily meditation practices. He rises very early and begins his day with guided meditation audios. From the conversations I've had with him since he started this practice he seems to find a greater sense of peace and he says he feels less fearful when he meditates. He still experiences anxiety about the unknowns (dad's always had to have definitive answers to everything) and he says he has at times uttered the 'why me?' prayer to God. God apparently hasn't yet answered that question, but dad does feel there's a reason for everything and feels the reason for this disease in his life at this time will be revealed to him as he begins to understand it, to heal it or to come to peace with it. Communing with God through meditation, says dad, makes him feel better and less afraid and sometimes clearer answers will come in the stillness of meditation.

I don't think it matters how we talk to God. And I've not seen any evidence that piety in prayer has gotten me more divine intervention than my raw, real and gritty prayers. I've had more than a harsh word or two to say to God and my angels about bringing cancer into my dad's life. But as upset as I've been sometimes, somewhere deep inside I trust we will be guided with grace and wherever it leads it will be to a 'a place where we'll be safe.'

What a Wonderful World

The colours of the rainbow so pretty in the sky
Are also on the faces of people going by
I see friends shaking hands saying how do you do
They're really saying I love you.
I hear babies cry, I watch them grow
They'll learn much more than I'll ever know
And I think to myself what a wonderful world
Yes I think to myself what a wonderful world.

('What a wonderful world' — *Louis Armstrong*)

In apartheid South Africa, for people of colour, life was far from wonderful. Yes, we had the 'trees of green' and 'clouds of white'. In fact, you'd be hard pressed to find a more beautiful landscape than Cape Town with its majestic Table Mountain. But the ugliness of racial hatred and segregation tainted it all and left a cloud of pain hovering over the majority of its people. But the old Chinese proverb 'better to light a candle than to curse the darkness' was as true then as it is now. Those 'candles' took the form of simple things in our community — enjoying music, song, dance, food and having fun together.

And, for all his seriousness and sternness, dad was a facilitator of many fun times in our lives. He was out on the streets with us and the neighbourhood children playing games; hours spent playing skaloulo (a running ball game), or kennetjie (a hitting game where a stump is placed on two bricks and one team or person has to hit it as far as possible). Sometimes he even got into five stones, a game played mainly by girls but some boys tried to give us a run for our money.

(In the game, five stones were tossed on the hands of players, ending when one person was left with stones on their hand). I used to get teased about my witches fingers because my hands and fingers were long and bony even then. But they were great hands for tossing and holding onto five stones — I fast became one of the better players in our neighbourhood. We used to tease my dad about his stumpy hands and short, stubby fingers, but he could out toss me from time to time.

Dad was also one of the many who played tennis with us on the street. He'd help us carry our buckets or tins of sand and draw out the sand lines of the tennis court in the street. He went easy on the girls and some of the younger kids. But when he got into the matches with my brothers, it was a case of all guns blazing. None of them would give an inch and they'd be out there slogging for victory in the hot summer sun. Both my brothers are good at their sport and I believe they gained their competitive streak from their days with dad on the makeshift courts and running tracks in the neighbourhood streets.

We ran sprinting races, relays and mini marathons around the neighbourhood blocks and more times than not dad would be right there with us either running the races or, on the pavement, cheering the teams on.

We didn't have time to be bored. There were too many games and activities going on in the streets and backyards. It would be long past nightfall before the sounds of the last games died down. One by one the kids from each home would respond to their mothers' calls to come in for dinner, but that was usually after the third or fourth call or when the dads were sent out to get us. On the odd occasion, dad would get in on a game with us out on the street and then mum would have to come out to get us and him. It was usually pitch dark by then.

Within the walls of our home there were rarely moments of silence. Tunes were regularly belting from the old record player and dad would whistle or sing along to Elvis Presley, Cliff Richard, The Beatles, Louis Armstrong, Frank Sinatra and many more.

And my parents would not only dance the jive or rock and roll, they would sometimes teach us some moves. In my early childhood and teen years I was the worst dancer amongst my siblings and often teased about taking after dad (he's no Fred Astaire). But mum is our Ginger Rogers. These days when we get together and dance, she's still got rhythm and cool moves on the floor. To his credit, dad never let his awkwardness on the dance floor stop him from taking his turn at a waltz, a jive or even a bit of rhythmic soul moves. He's not one to worry about what others think of him and he doesn't mind having a laugh at himself either. And I love how he'd take his daughters for a turn around the floor when we were going through partnerless phases and turned up solo for family or community functions.

Dominoes, poker and klaverjas were games that brought players from other streets, neighbourhoods and even Franciscan presbyteries into our home. The competition was fierce and little or no grace was given — not even to the novices or priests. Their collars or brown robes tied at the waist with a rope belt counted for naught when they sat around the dining room table competing in a card game or playing dominoes. The house would ring with bantering, laughter, not to mention their various tactics to psych each other out. We kids were allowed to play with the grown ups and we gave them a run for their money. Dad had taught us how to play most of the games at a very young age and we could certainly hold our own against most of the adults. No prizes were offered. Just outsmarting dad at some of these games was considered a victory of great magnitude.

Summer was a time filled with picnics, barbecues and beach trips. Sometimes there'd be up to ten families in our group descending on the popular parks or beaches. Out would come the cricket bats and ball, badminton sets, volleyball sets and soccer balls; everyone got involved in a game. Our summer outings were not for those who simply wanted to lie around getting a suntan. We played 'chasey' with dad and for a guy with short legs he had some speed. It was only when we got to the later childhood years that we could catch up to him. Dad's multi-coloured swimsuit was a source of great teasing from us and so was his hairstyle. Dad was already going bald at a young age, but used to comb a longer tuft of hair over his bald patch. When he'd be out in the pools or ocean swimming the piece of hair would move back and forth as he turned his face sideways for air. Even from a distance we could always pinpoint dad in the water by his multi coloured swimsuit and the waving of his hair 'vlaggie' (little flag).

Christmas and New Year's Eve were the two big celebrations in our family and community. On Christmas Eve we were sent to bed early for a few hours sleep and then would be woken around 10pm. We would go with mum and dad to church — there were carols by candlelight and then midnight mass. If we were good in church, we were allowed to open our Christmas presents after midnight mass — and it probably was what led us to be on our best behaviour. If our neighbours were awake in the early hours of the morning, we'd all go around to wish them 'merry Christmas'. We usually had only a few hours sleep because Christmas morning was a bubble of excitement as we prepared Christmas lunch — a feast of hams, chicken, pork, potato salad, green salad, steamed vegetables, roast potatoes and sauces. With the range of desserts on offer too, I still wonder how we managed to fit so much food into our bellies. But there was no way anyone in my family was going to pass up on trifle or Christmas pudding with hot custard. Dad can still out gobble the rest of us — for years he's had a paunch that makes him look like he's about four months pregnant. His take on this — it's taken him years to cultivate his paunch, so he has to keep it happy.

New Year's Eve would often start with a barbecue. Dad was and still is 'Mr Barbecue' — in his place behind the grill with tongs in hand flipping meat, chicken and sausage. His sampling and tasting as he goes is done only because it has to be cooked to perfection. He is brilliant at the barbecue and I've yet to find someone who can cook up meat the way he does, so even though we know he's going to sample a few pieces of meat along the way, we're happy to leave him in charge of all barbecuing.

New Year's Eve or New Year's Day wouldn't be a celebration without song or dance. Apart from dancing the night away with family and friends, dad would sometimes take us into Cape Town city to watch the 'klopse'. These are music or dance bands who dress in colourful costumes and perform cultural songs. The music and performances are so vibrant and filled with such humour you'd either be shaking with laughter or tapping your feet to the rhythmic sounds.

This was certainly not a dark time of year. In fact, for most of the year, I marvelled at how mum and dad managed to keep us from 'cursing the darkness' in a place like South Africa. We were always aware of the danger, anger and fear. But our world was made brighter by parents who found and welcomed joy, laughter, music, song and good friends. And the boy in dad was never far away when it came to having fun with his children. Our world with him became 'a wonderful world.'

Hard to Say Goodbye to Yesterday

I don't know where this road
Is going to lead
All I know is where we've been
And what we've been through.
If we get to see tomorrow
I hope it's worth all the wait
It's so hard to say goodbye to yesterday.
And I'll take with me the memories
To be my sunshine after the rain
It's so hard to say goodbye to yesterday.

('Hard to say goodbye to yesterday' — *Boyz II Men*)

I don't know too many people who can say they enjoy goodbyes. There's nothing easy about them. Endings are hard, no doubt, but I think beginnings are even harder. The unfamiliar and unknown always makes us anxious. My family's was no different.

My parents' decision to leave South Africa and start a new life with the family in a new country came many years before we actually left. Dad started applying for immigration to Australia when I was close to twelve years old. We finally got the nod when I was twenty. The most valuable lesson I learned through my father's tenacity was to never give up. We always knew when the rejection letters came from the Australian embassy because it was written all over dad's face. But, year after year, when he had no reason to believe the answer would be any different he found the guts to continue applying. It is often his strength, courage and sheer persistence that I think about when I've pursued my own seemingly unreachable dreams. More often than not, I've found that what once seemed impossible becomes a reality by simply never, ever giving up.

Though dad never wavered from the decision to leave South Africa, I know it was probably one of the hardest ones he's ever had to make. He wanted to be part of the solution in South Africa, not someone who ran from the problem. But in the end the safety and wellbeing of his family was paramount; more vital to him than the pursuit of freedom for a troubled and dangerous land.

As we approached our teen years, the political unrest became more volatile in South Africa. Stray bullets from police gunfire in areas of unrest took many an innocent life. On more than one occasion, our school bus had to ride through burning tyres and stone-throwing crowds. These were wild times in South Africa. The tides were slowly turning and the oppressed black people were rising up against the injustices they'd lived with for decades. We had no idea how long it would take nor how many lives would be lost before the desired 'freedom' of a suppressed nation was achieved. But we knew that there'd be no rest or peace until a majority black nation was no longer suppressed by a white minority ruling group.

In 1985, in my final year of high school, there was daily violence and unrest had reached a fever pitch and students became more and more involved in political protests than attending school. The South African Board of Education closed all coloured schools but issued memos that we were still expected to sit the final exams. And so began the clandestine activities of secret meetings or finding our way to teachers' homes to get some kind of tutoring and preparation for the final exams.

It was one of the most stressful times of my life. I spent nights with my head buried in the little material I was able to obtain, desperately trying to get ready for the finals. I cried myself to sleep at nights because I was so uncertain of everything and so anxious about the possibility of failure. The violence was out of control and martial law was enforced. Army and police officers were everywhere and curfews meant everyone had to be off the streets by 8pm.

It was dad who drove me to and from the Goodwood showgrounds — the rendezvous point for transport to the exam. We were picked up by bus and escorted by armed soldiers to a military base. I wrote all my final high school exams in an airport hangar on a military base, surrounded by armed soldiers. And, though I knew he worried the whole time, dad encouraged me to do my best, to stay focused on the exam questions and to not be afraid. I wished I could take that worry away. Still I was grateful for his presence in the car every day as we drove to and from the pick-up and drop-off points.

After the many rejections we'd seen for immigration to Australia over nearly a decade, I don't think we really expected a 'yes'. So, when we finally received that letter of acceptance in 1986, it came as a shock. I was in my first year of a BA degree at university. The youngest sibling in our family was twelve years old. And dad was at the pinnacle of his career, finally in a position where he was starting to see the fruits of his very long labour. His bosses held him in high regard and he was being offered more opportunities, perks and incentives (unusual given the social and professional segregation of the times). But dad's employers were liberal-minded and he had done a lot to guide and influence their views and work practices towards a more integrated and fair approach.

When I think of what he, and so many good people like him, sacrificed in leaving South Africa, I'm filled with intense sadness and equally intense anger. I feel dad was on the brink of something momentous in his professional life. He'd come such a long way for a boy who'd been parentless from such a young age, raised in an orphanage in his early childhood, wandered the streets in his youth. I felt he deserved the same good fortune Oliver Twist got to experience with his benefactor, Mr Brownlow.

The months before we left Cape Town were a whirlwind; medical checks, packing, selling, a twenty-first birthday party for my oldest brother and farewell parties. I don't think the reality of saying goodbye to people we'd grown up with and were unlikely to ever see again hit until the morning of 16 January 1987. It was only as we were hugging and kissing through teary embraces that the reality of the ending and the daunting prospect of a new beginning hit home.

And then, not only was it the first time any of us had been on a plane, but we had a long fifteen-hour flight to Hong Kong to contend with. We hardly noticed that we were 'flight virgins'. We were far too sad at having to say goodbye to what we knew and far too anxious about the unknown in Australia to pay much attention to the aircraft, its staff or the other passengers.

Usually, when I'm in such sorrow, I veer towards something familiar to comfort me. But this time there was nothing familiar about the journey ahead, save the presence of my parents and siblings. And we were as grief-stricken as each other to be of any great comfort to one another.

As the plane angled and turned away from Cape Town I caught one last glimpse of Table Mountain. I couldn't stop the tears from spilling over. I glanced around at my dad and what I saw on his face only mirrored the heartache within me. He'd trampled through many of its rugged paths, walking out his angst from his life's challenges and I know that mountain was his sanctuary for so many years. As the plane climbed higher and higher and the mountain became smaller and, finally, disappeared all he had were his memories to be 'the sunshine after the rain' as we picked up speed racing towards an unknown land and life. And I know that he felt every bit of that hard goodbye to his yesterdays.

Hero

And then a hero comes along
With the strength to carry on
And you cast your fears aside
And you know you can survive
So when you feel like hope is gone
Look inside you and be strong
And you finally see the truth
That a hero lies in you

('Hero' — *Mariah Carey*)

These days, when we think of heroes, we tend to look to our sporting stars, our political leaders and our entertainment celebrities. Seems like you're only acknowledged as a hero of sorts when you're given the public nod for a deed that's blasted over television, Twitter or Facebook.

But there are so many people who go about their every day ordinary lives in extraordinary ways never getting the acknowledgement they deserve. They're not going to get the Victoria Cross for bravery or the Nobel Peace prize, yet the consistency of their actions and their persistence through life's challenges transforms the lives of their family and community. Yet when I think how one transformed life transforms another and another, I wonder why so many in our world go through life as unsung heroes. My dad's one of them. And I've not seen more of the hero come out in him than through the first few years of arrival in Australia.

Though we had all, throughout the oppressive years in apartheid South Africa, longed for the freedom that life offered in Australia, when it was within our grasp, we didn't know what to do with it. For some time after landing in Australia my mother and my siblings and I were emotional messes. The dark clouds of oppression and inferiority still hung around our lives. When I'd travel with my cousin into Melbourne during our first few weeks in Australia, I'd look for the signs on buses and trains to tell me where I had to sit or stand. My dad's sister and her family had been in Australia about five years by the time we arrived so they'd long moved on from life in South Africa.

My cousin had to remind me a few times that I was no longer in South Africa and I could travel in any carriage on any train and stand or sit anywhere on the buses and trams. That was only a small challenge I faced. Everything was different, but we weren't. We still carried the wounds and ingrained thought patterns from our former life. And that made it difficult to integrate into our new life. Added to that was the homesickness. I never thought we'd be homesick for a country whose politics had scourged our people and left us tainted with some bitter memories. But I missed the people we left behind and I missed that mountain — beautiful Table Mountain that greets you from every angle of Cape Town as she looms over the city in her majestic glory. Each one of us went through tears, feelings of wanting to return to South Africa and anxiety about never being able to fit in, in Australia. Mum's blood pressure was at unhealthy levels from sadness, anxiety and worrying about her children's unhappiness.

Dad's serious side came to the fore (even went up a few notches) and I don't remember him smiling much in the first two years of our life in Australia. He had to find work, a new home for his family and cope with our sorry, sad faces for months on end.

Yet, not once did I hear him complain. He'd just go about being the rock of Gibraltar to all of us. But he hardly smiled and he seemed to age overnight. Money was tight; after paying for our tickets over to Australia, there was not much left from the proceeds of selling the house in South Africa.

We did have enough for a deposit on a small new home and, as I watched him struggle to recreate a decent life for his family, I often wondered if he regretted leaving South Africa. After all he'd reached the point where he was earning enough to provide more opportunities for all of us. While we may have had to contend with excessive fear and anxiety back in South Africa, his career success would've meant a few more doors opening for us as a family.

I never spoke to him about what he felt during that time. But I could imagine how hard it would have been to start at the bottom of the professional pile and rebuild his career. And live with a stressed out wife and five unhappy children. I could feel his anxiety even though he put on a brave face and continued to plod up that very steep hill of challenges in a new country. I do remember him being sick a few times. He would often end up with severe stomach pain and vomiting. It wasn't food poisoning or anything like that as we'd all eat the same food and none of us were ill. I do believe it was excessive anxiety that just wound him up in knots and made it difficult for him to keep his food down at times. Not that it stopped him in the least from getting through each difficult day. He just never stopped trying to make things work.

I don't think dad's even aware of how much strength he exhibited through that time and how much his rock solid consistency held our family together and slowly turned things onto a more positive road for all of us. In his awkward, emotionally-challenged way he managed to nurture my mum through her anxiety and fears and he helped us, his children, to adapt to the culture in Australia. I wanted to finish my university degree, but I knew my parents couldn't afford even the miniscule university fees at the time, so I found a part-time job at a Mexican restaurant and waitressed my way through university. And dad was my chauffeur to and from work a few nights a week. He'd sit up and wait for my call which at times was as late as midnight and come out in the cold and dark to collect me from the restaurant. And that was apart from driving my brothers to and from their part-time jobs too. Dad's always encouraged us to fend for ourselves and earn our own money from a young age, but he's always been a constant beacon shining just enough light for us to find our way through the shadows of untrodden paths. If at times we needed hand-holding along the rocky roads, he was always the first one to extend a steady hand.

I still hurt when I think of what dad sacrificed to give his family a better life. I still wish he could've gotten it all in the country of his birth. He's often expressed the wish that he'd like his ashes scattered on Table Mountain when he passes over, so I know it's still the place he loves most in the world. As cancer now looms with its greedy deathlike tentacles in his life, I can't get my mind around a journey I may have to take in the future to fulfil his wish. I also miss that mountain some days, but I don't want to see it again if I have to trade my father's life to gaze upon its magnificent vista.

I'm counting on the journey ahead as dad faces cancer to dig up even more of the hero I saw in him as he built a new life in a country that was so new and so unfamiliar to him. I'm counting on the same perseverance I saw in him as he continued to rise each morning weary from anxiety and bruised to the core from the sadness in his family and still do what needed to be done to feed and shelter his family.

I'm counting on dad to continue to be the hero in our lives, for he has earned that title many times over every time he's cast his fears aside and done what had to be done for his family to survive and thrive. The hero has always been within him.

The way we were

Memories, may be beautiful and yet
what's too painful to remember
we simply choose to forget
so it's the laughter we will remember
whenever we remember
the way we were.

('The way we were' — *Barbra Streisand*)

Time heals the deepest of wounds and even if they're never fully healed time certainly knows how to soothe and scab them over so they're bearable to live with. It was time and a genuine focus on making the most of our new life in Australia that slowly, but surely eased the pain of leaving behind our loved ones.

We weren't ready to let go of them completely and the first few years were spent on long distance phone calls and hours of card and letter writing. Sometimes I was sure I spent more times writing novel-like letters to my friends than on my studies. I outlined every detail of what I was up to and taught them Aussie slang and expressions through pages of writing. In return I insisted on every bit of gossip and details of who was up to what with whom. Of all the members in our family dad was the one who probably stayed in touch the least with the ones we'd left behind. He was fully focused on creating the new life in Australia and would occasionally ring the siblings or friends he'd left behind.

Dad's the one who stayed steady and strong through the earlier months in Australia, doing what he had to do to help us adjust. Within two years we'd all made the adjustment and our friendship horizons were broadening by the year. Yet dad hasn't found the same type of friendships he had in South Africa. He's met people through mum (husbands of her friends) and he continued to bond with people he'd known back in South Africa who also migrated to Australia, but he's not found the deep bond he shared with the two recovering alcoholics, who'd filled our home with such humour and such raw and gritty tales. I'm not sure if it's a conscious choice to keep himself shielded. Since his history has shown him that eventually he ends up saying goodbye to the people he lets into his heart it's possible he's chosen to keep people at a healthy distance. Maybe he was just too busy trying to build a new life for his family that he didn't take the time to get to know too many new people, let alone bond with them. Or maybe it's none of these reasons and he's simply chosen to be more of a loner than he was before. Dad's always been a complex man so I couldn't begin to unravel all the reasons behind the things he's done or choices and decisions he's made. I've wondered over the last few years why he didn't actively seek out the kind of friendships he once had. I've wondered if he's ever felt lonely or starved of deep friendship. It's one thing to be surrounded and loved by your family, but that often comes with its own baggage and agendas. Sometimes friends just bring a perspective and insight into life that's free of all the family history and expectations. And that allows a growth that's not stunted by the stranglehold of family 'must or should do's.' I often wish dad had more friends with similar interests to his, but I'm conscious that he might not wish that for himself. He's certainly always been content with his own company.

I did notice the storytelling of his younger years became more prominent in Australia. The tales of his childhood in the orphanage, his teen years running around on the streets, his young adult years hiking up Table Mountain and his friendships became a regular feature around the dining table a few years after we'd settled into life in Australia. He had shared some of them in bygone years in South Africa, but we heard more of them after we'd been in Australia a few years. Maybe it was his way of trying to preserve the memories of those good ole days or hanging onto the way things were in our old life.

The other way we tried to hang onto the familiar of the past was to seek out other ex- South Africans. Most of the people we socialised with in those early years were people we met through dad's family who'd already been in Australia for five years or people we'd known over there who had also migrated here. But as time went by we realised that it often made it more challenging to integrate into Australian culture, so we slowly started seeking out different cultural experiences.

Outside our social circles we started to meet people from other cultures. Dad started meeting Asian, Australian and other ethnic groups through his working life, us kids started doing the same through our university and school life and mum joined some spiritual and women's groups and started broadening her cultural horizons that way.

It took a while to get used to some of the expressions and mannerisms unique to the different cultures, but now we use them as though they've always been a part of our lives. I found the Aussie greeting of 'g'day mate' rather odd at first. I couldn't understand why they used it morning, noon and night, when the 'g'day' clearly implied day time, and I felt rather weird being called 'mate.' These days it rolls off my tongue as though it's been part of my vernacular since a toddler.

There were a few things in the Aussie version of English dad encouraged us not to use as he insisted on 'proper' English as we'd been taught in South Africa. He would cringe at the Aussie colloquial use of 'but' at the end of a sentence. The locals would describe a scenario and then end with 'but' usually as some sort of inflection and we'd be waiting for the qualifying sentence that usually followed 'but.' It never came. With time we realised it was merely an inflection in their description or narration. We were never encouraged by dad to adopt it though in our speech nor to take on the Aussie pronunciation of the letter 'H.' Saying 'haitch' for the letter 'H' is common practice in Australia, but to this day we pronounce 'H' as aitch. I'm doing the same thing now to my twelve-year-old daughter, insisting on 'aitch' instead of 'haitch.' Sometimes she gets irritated with me for correcting her, but I'm a stickler for some things in English as much as dad's been all these years. There are some things of the way we were that will continue to form part of what we are now and will still become.

Apart from being a great healer, time does not stand still. It moves all things and all people along, no matter how much they might want to stand still and stay locked in a time capsule. We noticed the responses to our calls and letters to loved ones in South Africa slowed as the years went by. While we still missed them and they us, time and life moved forward. New experiences replaced the old ones whether we planned them or not. As we began to let go of the way things were and became more open to the new life in Australia we started creating new memories — ones that were less painful, filled with hope and free of oppression and danger. It was a lot easier to recreate these kinds of memories over and over again because they felt good.

When dad started telling more and more of the stories in his earlier life around the dining table he always told it with humour and little or no regret. Sometimes I'd wonder how he could laugh at some of the tragedies and challenges he'd been through. As we've created new memories in Australia and we retell some of those to my daughter, along with the old ones of our life in South Africa I notice dad still tells most of the stories with such animation and humour. Sometimes it's hard to believe we've lived through such challenges, because there's so much laughter around the memories. And then I realise he's probably just choosing to forget the pain and to 'remember the laughter' whenever he remembers 'the way we were.'

Satisfied Mind

Money can't buy back your youth when you're old
A friend when you're lonely, oh, peace to your soul
The wealthiest person is a pauper at times
Compared to the man with a satisfied mind

('Satisfied Mind' — *Jeff Buckley*)

I often heard the 'money is the root of all evil' phrase come out of dad's mouth when I was younger. I can't say I understood exactly what it meant at that young age, but with the way mum and dad used to fight about money I figured there had to be some truth in it. It's only years later as I grew into adulthood that I've come to understand that money per se is not the root of anything, including evil. It's just something we use to trade with. Our mindset and relationship to money — well that's a whole other story. Greed is the root of most evils and it's not a tangible thing like money that we can see or touch, but it sure brings a powerful energy to how money is used or not used.

I think dad's use of the phrase 'money is the root of all evil' may have stemmed from doctrines and thought patterns passed on through his years in the catholic orphanage and growing up in poverty. It's possible that the lack of money may have felt evil to him at times. Sometimes in life when we're unable to attain something, we can end up knocking it or taking an 'it doesn't matter' attitude. But I believe that anyone who says money doesn't matter is either delusional or not totally honest with themselves. And I've not found a better description of the impact of poverty than that shared by Harry Potter author JK Rowling in her Commencement Address at the Harvard Alumni Association in 2008. She stated that 'poverty entails fear, and stress, and sometimes depression; it means a thousand petty humiliations and hardships. Climbing out of poverty by your own efforts, that is indeed something on which to pride yourself, but poverty itself is romanticised only by fools.' And since she's experienced the extremes of not having and having money, I'd say she has a pretty good grasp on the concept of poverty.

Though dad may have said money and evil in the same sentence more times than once, I don't believe he truly believed that. He spent a lot of energy over the years trying to improve his financial standing. He went to night school to gain qualifications to improve his opportunities for earning a better wage. He always sought out extra duties at work other than those assigned to his job description to be a contribution to his colleagues and to open up further opportunities. And to this day he still buys weekly lottery tickets. So whatever he may have said about money, he was definitely always trying to make more.

On the flip side though, dad never let an abundance of money or lack thereof dictate his interactions with others. He was himself, warts and all with company executives who had loads of money and the same with the labourers in the quarry struggling to make ends meet. He was not intimidated by those more financially successful than he was because he didn't believe it made them a better or worse person than he was. In later years we'd talk about how people related to and with money. And dad and I would often agree that money would likely enhance more of what you truly are as a person. People who were stingy, unkind and lacking in generosity by nature were not going to suddenly become giving, kind and generous if they suddenly came into a huge sum of money. Chances are they'd become more of the negative qualities because their fears would only increase. There'd be bigger sums of money to lose and therefore bigger fears around losing it.

In our household there was mostly just enough money to pay the bills, take care of the necessities and occasionally enjoy a few luxuries. Birthdays and Christmas were the treat times of year when something special was bought in the way of gifts and clothes. Every year, just before Christmas mum and dad would take us five kids into town to do our annual clothes shopping. That's when we usually got the supply of underwear, socks, clothes and shoes which had to last us the entire year. We'd walk up and down Adderley Street in Cape Town stopping in the various department and shoe stores. It was the time of year dad hated the most and he was always grumpy. Apart from not being thrilled about having to spend all that money in one hit, he and I would invariably end up in an argument or a battle of wills. I liked to look at many shops before deciding what I wanted. He hated the 'trying on different styles' process. I truly believe it was the most torturous thing I put him through. And I often chose what I wanted from the first one or two shops we'd gone through. He couldn't believe I'd make him walk up and down the streets of Cape Town only to go back to the first shops to get what I liked. By the time I was in my early teens he'd hand me a sum of money and tell me to meet him at a designated point in a couple of hours with my gear in hand. And if I didn't have everything I want — too bad. He wasn't having it — we left and I had to make do with what I'd found.

Gift-giving cost money and mum always had stylish taste so she'd want to choose nice gifts for family and friends. It invariably led to fights with dad because she often exceeded the budget he'd set for gifts. I can't remember too many festive seasons when there wasn't a fight in the household between mum and dad. Christmas day in and of itself was fabulous and we always had joyous celebrations. But the weeks preceding it — well there was definitely not 'peace on earth' in our home.

I believe the fear of not having enough money to support his family was the driving factor underneath dad's consistent desire to keep tight controls on the budget and spending. And underneath that I'm sure were the harsh reminders of poverty he'd grown up with. Yet despite these fears, he found his joys and pleasures in simple things.

Dad isn't one to be enchanted by grand houses, fancy cars and designer labels. He dresses simply and comfortably and favours clothes that support his love of the outdoors. He loves hanging around in his overalls and track suits, pottering around in the garden. In fact he loves his track suits so much he's often tried to go out in them, but mum has often halted those plans with a nag about changing into appropriate attire. He's done it, but not without protest or grumbling. There's been the odd occasion when he's ignored her nagging and gone out in the same clothes he's been wearing out in the garden — grubby stains and all.

Dad's driven very practical, economical cars over the years — usually station wagons or cars big enough to transport his wife and five children. The car he loved the most was an old, dodgy looking pickup truck he used to call 'Turbie.' I can't remember how many times we had to get behind 'Turbie' while dad pushed from the front holding the steering wheel and then jumping into it when it spluttered to life. He'd wave with a grin on his face and drive old 'Turbie' down the road before disappearing, often in a cloud of smoke, around the corner.

The homes dad's been drawn the most to, were not the fancy, palace-like mansions some of his bosses or more affluent friends owned. He'd admire them and offer his congratulations for their achievements and success. But it was the homes filled with lively games, laughter, music, good food and more often than not much, much smaller than the big mansions that dad would be most at home in. Anywhere where camaraderie and friendship were the dominant adornments is where you'd find my dad fitting in like a well-worn pair of slippers.

Though dad's bank balances have not had many zeroes tacked on, he has been most content with things like mum's amazing home-cooking, the company of his children and grandchild, the banter with one or two good friends, pottering around in his garden and nature and beachside walks and hikes. Great monetary fortunes have not graced his life, but enduring blessings have and these satisfied his mind. And he is the richer for it.

Sunrise, Sunset

Sunrise, Sunset
Sunrise, Sunset
Swiftly fly the years
One season following another
Laden with happiness and tears
What words of wisdom can I give them?
How can I help to ease their way?

('Sunrise, sunset' — from *Fiddler on the roof*)

Every experience in life has its sunrise and sunset, but I think the hardest sunset any parent ever faces is the one of letting go their children. Parents teeter between stepping back to allow the adult to emerge in the child or crossing the line and protecting the child from some of the harsher adult experiences. My daughter's only twelve years old, but these days they seem to hanker for independence far earlier than we did, and I find myself teetering often.

As his first four children started moving towards adult independence (the youngest was still in high school), dad encouraged us to know about finances: household expenses, budgets and enough income to support any lifestyle we chose. All of us had been working part-time or after school jobs since we were in our early teens and dad's emphasis was always on trying to save as much as we could.

By the time I'd reached twenty-one I had enough money saved for my own car. Dad helped by scrutinising the automobile section of the *Trading Post*, local newspapers and car yards until we found my brown Nissan Bluebird — the ugliest, muddy brown colour and really not much to look at but I was enamoured with that car. It meant greater independence but was also, thanks to dad's checking, a solid, reliable car and not just my means to freedom.

Dad was the one who taught me to drive in South Africa, though I failed my driver's test the first time. I'd expected to flunk on the hills of Green Point because as much as dad coaxed, showed and even yelled the coordinating moves I needed to stay on the hill without stalling, I struggled to get it right.

In the end it wasn't the hills that got me; my undoing was a motorcyclist whom I almost hit as I swerved out of a parking spot without checking the mirrors properly. We were close to leaving South Africa at that time so I decided to try again once we reached Australia. I was so disappointed with myself after that first test I lost my nerve and needed some time before giving it another go. But I'd also figured out (like most daughters) that dads are not always the best ones to teach us how to drive.

We'd been in Australia just over two years when my sister and I were ready to fly the nest. We'd been out clubbing for about six months, met a bunch of people we thought were cool at the time and also taken a fancy to some guys. But my parents had very strict rules about bringing guys home — well they didn't mind the bringing them home part, but they weren't going to allow anything more than a 'hang around on the couch' situation. Mum would hover, constantly offering a drink or food. Dad would just come in and sit down amongst us and our friends, even if it occurred to him that we might want privacy. He wasn't the type to indulge us at his own expense of missing the news or a favourite TV show. He's always done exactly what he wanted, but I'd bet that sometimes he'd intrude on our 'friend hangout' time just to annoy us. He had that kind of twisted humour.

My sister and I had been planning to move out together for a while and started looking at furniture and other household items. We were excited, but we hadn't bargained on mum's reaction. Our announcement of our plans ended in an argument with mum — the details are vague — but I suspect it had something to do with her not being ready to let us go and being unresponsive and less than enthusiastic about our moving out. Being young adults and focused on what we wanted, we handled the situation with a lot less sensitivity than we could have. We were pretty obstinate and aggressive young women at the time and the final result was not only the big fight with mum but then dad promptly kicking us out of home. I don't think he really had a problem with us being ready or wanting to move out of home, but he did have a problem with us upsetting mum that way and being so brash. So we had to manifest a home a bit earlier than planned and for a while things were very uncomfortable between us and my parents. But as soon as we needed help with setting up our household and gardening tasks, he was the first one over to help us out.

It wasn't long after moving out that I met my daughter's father — an African American basketball player. He was eleven years older than me and had a two-year-old son. But, he also had the reputation as a ladies' man (as did his fellow basketball players). Dad let me know in no uncertain terms that he didn't approve of that relationship. I'd spent years being the studious, diligent girl always focused on school and university and I was ready to spread my wings once I'd graduated and experience some excitement. The older man with the prominent and exciting athletic career represented that to me. Plus I'd always been a bit headstrong (a lot like dad in fact, though neither one of us would've admitted that at the time).

Our relationship took a nose dive — so far down in fact that we stopped talking to each other for a year. In so many ways I felt lost without dad during that time and I can't remember the number of times I wanted to reach out and make up with him, but stubborn pride kept us from each other. It was a long, long year and most times I'd cry quietly in the car after visiting mum because dad would usually walk out when I arrived. I can't remember now how we made up — I suppose it's not important, but when we did, I was so grateful to have him back in my life. Dad may have wished otherwise at times because it wasn't long after that when the tumultuous roller coaster began with my boyfriend. I'm sure dad detested that time of my life. My boyfriend and I split and reconciled a number of times over the following years and dad was always the one helping me move away and then back to our home.

Now, as a parent, I can see what that might have meant and can't believe dad didn't grab me and throttle some sense into me. He never interfered again in my relationship, but would just help me out without a word. The only protest he ever made about moving me back and forth so many times was over the amount of shoes he had to move each time (I acquired many pairs during my twenties, earning dad's nickname of Imelda Marcos).

The relationship with my boyfriend ended for good when I was four months pregnant. Dad's only comment was to tell me to come home, where I spent the remaining months of my pregnancy. It is where I began the long, healing journey under their nurturing care. I expected 'I told you so' from dad. I expected long lectures about how foolish I'd been, but I got none of that. He knew my soul was scarred and spirit shattered and he wasn't going to add salt to my deep, blistering wounds. He helped me get the house on the market and advised me all the way through on how to best come out of the situation with as little collateral damage as possible.

The greatest gift he gave me though was tactile healing through back and foot massages. We didn't speak much during those months, not about my broken relationship anyway. He knew I needed time to process what I'd just been through and to find a way to heal from it so I could be ready for the arrival of my baby. It was one of the few times in my life that dad didn't offer many words of wisdom, yet he helped ease the way just by being there for me and caring for me through his actions. In so many ways he's often been the sunrise which has followed the sunset of many of my life's experiences.

Be a clown

Be a clown, be a clown,
All the world loves a clown.
Act a fool, play the calf,
And you'll always have the last laugh

('Be a clown' *— Judy Garland and Gene Kelly)*

Humour is the balm which soothed many of the challenges our family went through in our birth country, South Africa and our adopted country, Australia. Despite his very serious personality, dad was often at the centre of the family's funny experiences. He has the uncanny knack of doing goofy things, in a most serious way. He rarely sees how funny he's being; made even more so by being very serious as he explains why he thought his actions were a good idea at the time.

Not long after we'd arrived in Australia dad discovered the delights of the 'trash and treasure' markets. The biggest delight was savings he was making having 'another man's trash, his treasure', spending hours on Sunday mornings at markets, scoping them for useful second-hand objects for the household or his children.

My youngest sister was still in high school for a few years after our arrival in Australia and she had a distance to walk to school with a very heavy school bag. One Sunday dad came home with an excited and proud look on his face as he presented her with an old bike he'd found at the Sunday market. The bike was so ragged it elicited nothing more than disdain from my sister. But dad was not deterred; there was more. He presented her with his second gift — a wheelie shopping cart like ones we'd see old people manoeuvring around the supermarkets. His bright idea? My sister could connect this old cart to the back of the raggedy bike and have something to tow her school bag in. He was deeply pleased with himself.

My sister not only stared at him, eyebrows raised, but refused to go outside and watch him test-drive his brilliant idea. Again, he was not deterred. He connected the cart to the bike and was about to take off when he hit a snag. The wheel spokes were bent and some had come loose; that bike wasn't going anywhere, let alone towing a shopping cart. My sister, who had relented and come to watch, stomped off in frustration but promptly burst out laughing as she told the rest of the family the story. We fell on the floor laughing, tears streaming down our faces. Minutes later, dad appeared in the lounge room with a sheepish grin. He had, reluctantly no doubt, dumped his new found treasure with the rest of the trash in his garden trailer.

Not that the experience halted any other brilliant ways of saving money. Dad hasn't yet grasped the notion of 'penny wise and pound foolish'; he isn't committed to the thought that, in some instances, one must close the eyes to the price and spend in order to achieve long term gain.

Most people who know and love dad, know he's not a handyman. Trouble is — he doesn't know that (yet) or stubbornly refuses to accept the shortcoming. A few years after dad bought the house he and mum live in, it needed painting and retiling. Dad, deciding to take on the painting himself, did a reasonable job. He took his time; painted a room at a time.

When retiling the kitchen, however, things weren't quite as efficient. Dad had assembled a broom cupboard a few years earlier and it needed to be dismantled so that the floor tiles under it could be laid evenly. Surprisingly, he'd done an ok job of this cupboard which neatly housed the vacuum cleaner, mop, broom and other gadgets. The dismantling and reassembling of the broom cupboard seemed a good plan in theory, but, in his haste to complete the kitchen touch-ups and retiling, dad reassembled the cupboard when the tiling was done, and left out a wooden panel. The cupboard was skew and the doors wouldn't shut properly but he insisted that he'd done it right; got annoyed at us and mum for questioning him. Until, that was, he discovered the overlooked, but necessary panel in the yard. Tail between his legs, he had to dismantle the cupboard yet again and reassemble it — this time all the parts were in place before he secured it.

Dad had many ideas about how to get jobs done around the house — so many ways to make life comfortable for him and mum or save money that my sister coined the name 'ideas' man' for him. One of his more brilliant ideas was to make a little gardening bench (inspired, he said, by his days in the Catholic Church). Dad loves to potter in the garden, but the backyard is quite huge so he'd often end up with back pain from bending over to weed or plant. Dad remembered that the padded church pews had been reasonably comfortable for kneeling during long church rituals, so he decided to create something similar. A padded foot stool might have done the same job; they're big enough for kneeling and soft enough to keep the knees comfortable but dad probably wanted to save a buck again. He took the slats from an old bed, used carpet scraps, and filler from an old pillow as the padding and made the oddest creation I've laid eyes on. It looks as cheap and nasty as it is, but dad loves the little bench. And, by some great miracle, it has endured over the last few years. Dad can often be found pottering out in his backyard, that weird and warped looking bench not far away. It's been the subject of many family jokes, but he laughs along all the while clinging to the kneeling bench like vines to a trellis, and insisting it was one of his more brilliant ideas.

One incident that has become funny with time, though was definitely not at the time, involves dad's warped sense of punishment. It also involves my brother and an orange. When we were growing up in South Africa, mum would buy a certain amount of fruit each week and it was shared equally by the family. We weren't allowed to help ourselves to any food without asking. One particular week, mum hadn't yet divided out the oranges And, by day four or five, announced at the dining table that an orange had gone missing. Dad (using his most frightening gremlin face) cast his eyes around the table wanting to know who had taken the orange. All five children pleaded 'not guilty'. He sent us to our rooms and insisted there'd be no more food or playtime, until someone confessed.

A while later orange peels were discovered outside the bedroom window my two brothers shared. The youngest brother finally owned up. And the rest of us were relieved and though most of the time we five kids stuck together — we knew we would now get dinner and he'd be the one copping the ironing cord. That relief turned to dismay when dad announced that we all had to give our brother a whipping since his orange theft and failing to confess had resulted in all of us being banished to our rooms. We were mortified. To make matters worse, dad stood by and ensured we whipped our brother properly or else face our own whipping if we tried to go easy on him. My brother teases dad today about child abuse. His only response is to grin gleefully.

Though many times the driving intention behind some of our family experiences was serious, often, if things went awry, we found a touch of humour in it all. I'm sure that through our shared laughter we have been bound stronger and it had definitely increased our sense of happiness and intimacy. Laughter became the medicine that helped us swallow many bitter, harsh and challenging experiences. I think it kept us healthy, not only in body, but in mind and spirit too.

Dad was the lead clown. Though he never really set out to be one his often warped and goofy acts have been appreciated for many years. And thankfully he's not too serious and too stoic to appreciate that we love him more because of it and he often does 'have the last laugh' even if it is laughing at himself.

When a child is born

A ray of hope flitters in the sky
A shiny star lights up way up high
All across the land dawns a brand new morn
This comes to pass when a child is born.

('When a child is born' — *Johnny Mathis*)

Dad's first (and so far only) grandchild was born on 19 November 1997 at 11:42 am. I know the date and time well; I was the one who grunted, squeezed and pushed my way through five hours of labour to bring her forth. I'd like to say dad was there as a rock solid support through the labour, but he wasn't. My brother and then brother-in-law popped in when I was about half way through labour and disappeared as soon as a contraction hit and I started breathing deeply, loudly and bending over the bed. Mum and my youngest sister nurtured me through it. It really was a womanhood and sisterhood time, not so much by our choice, but because the men couldn't handle it.

As much as I'd have liked dad there, I didn't expect him to be. Dad's always been squeamish around blood or illness. And, I was born at home. When he was asked, to bury the placenta after I was delivered, he barely made it outside of the house before he was sick. He did get through it (burying my placenta) but not after a few bouts of nausea. Given that I'd heard this tale a few times in my life, I knew it would be asking for way to much to expect him to be at the birth of my daughter.

I had to have an episiotomy in the final moments of labour because the baby's heart rate started dropping and they wanted to get her out quickly. As a result I was on painkillers for a few days after the birth. And she was in intensive care due to respiratory problems. So I was stressed and dazed when dad arrived later in the day to see his granddaughter, but I remember the look on his face as though it happened yesterday.

My daughter has looked like different members in our family over the years, but the first person she looked like was dad. She had the same flat shape at the back of her head as dad; she had the same Obi-Wan Kenobi look of wisdom about her even as a newborn, that dad has. I'm not sure if it's because she resembled him or because she was tiny and helpless lying in the incubator in intensive care, but he was besotted from the moment he saw her. I'd never seen such tenderness in his face. The first thing he did was put his hand through the hole in the incubator and massaged her back. She stirred slightly at the touch of her grandpa's hands, but then continued to sleep soundly.

We'd already discovered that apart from her newborn looks, she was like dad when it came to food. Moments after she'd been born she was struggling to breathe, but that didn't stop her taking to the breast. She camped on each breast for fifteen minutes, guzzling down the first feed of colostrum as though it was her last meal. She'd struggle to breath throughout the first feed, but wouldn't detach from the breast. The nurse had to take her off both times so she could come up for air and breathe a little easier. When we told the story to the rest of the family and friends, the comments were mostly the same 'oh she already loves her food, just like her pa'. Dad would just grin like a Cheshire cat. We lived with mum and dad for at least four months after my daughter was born and it was a time when I revisited some of the more tender memories from my early childhood. It was also the time new and wonderful memories were created between my daughter and her grandparents. Much as he'd done with his children, dad loved the bath time routine with her; often singing the same old songs he sang to us at bath time. And he nurtured her with massage and gentle pats on the back. She always slept soundly in her grandpa's arms. At times he'd lie back on the couch and lay her on his chest, securely tucked into the crook of his arm and they'd both be sound asleep in seconds. She even resembled him in sleep — both their heads tilted similarly, chins pointing upwards and sleeping like the dead.

The strain and challenges of establishing ourselves in Australia were borne by dad, and showed in the extra lines, crevices even, on his face. Yet when my daughter was born, some of those lines disappeared. I saw him smiling more and slowly and steadily, tenderness crept not only into his face, but into his life. He was often the first one at the car when I'd pull up to visit my parents and would greet her with 'how's m'angel?' As she grew older he'd insist on his hugs from her and would say 'come give pa a propery hug' He was never content with just a quick cuddle from her and she would oblige with a big bear hug that lasted for more than a few seconds. She still does to this day (at twelve). She's idolised and adored her grandpa from day one and they share a very special bond. And I know she brought a new brightness to his life and soothed many of his past hurts with the limitless love she showered on him and he on her.

When I first heard 'dad has prostate cancer', apart from being in total shock and denial, my persistent thought was how to find the words to tell my daughter. I knew she would be devastated.

It was through a chat with dad that we decided he would tell her. I wasn't there when he did but from what he and mum said, it was the first time dad got teary since being diagnosed. And as I suspected she was devastated at the news and cried solidly for a while. Dad helped her to focus on the wonderful memories they've shared as pa and granddaughter and let her know they would go on to create many more memories together. Cancer was a serious illness, he explained, and then comforted her with his usual wisdom, saying it didn't necessarily mean death and that death could come in any way and it could come at any time for anyone no matter their age.

When I spoke with her later she was curled up against me crying and asking me 'why does it have to be my pa who has cancer? Why can't it be someone else's pa?' I had to remind her that it didn't matter whose pa it was, it was scary. Through her tears she said she was going to pray to the angels to keep her pa strong and to make him better. And I reminded her that if she continued to shower her pa with loads of love it would help make the journey ahead so much easier for him.

Her look through her tear stained face clearly said, 'Uh duh, mum', but then she leaned against me and simply said 'I love my pa so much and I'm only going to think good things for him.' And I realised that children continue to bring rays of hope through their untainted optimism and who knows — perhaps another 'brand new morn' will dawn for my dad just as it came to pass when his grandchild was born almost thirteen years ago.

Grandpa told me so

He said life is made for you to live
The best love is the love that you give
There'll be times when you wanna hold on but you gotta let go
And I live by those words 'cause Grandpa told me so.

('Grandpa told me so' — *Kenny Chesney*)

I think dad got to truly experience the giving and receiving of an almost pure and gentle love through the time and energy he put into his granddaughter. He gave us all — mum and his five children — the best love he could over the years, but sometimes it was mixed with fear, anger and the challenges from balancing being present and being out in the world trying to provide for us. By the time his granddaughter came into his life, he and mum had mellowed; their children were grown, had moved out of home and were supporting themselves. He had far less distracting him from being present to a new love in his life. Her own father (who left when I was four months pregnant) has had very inconsistent contact. And dad has been the most consistent father figure she's known. All the things little girls love doing with their daddies, she's done with her pa. She lapped up everything he taught her and everything she experienced with him.

It was dad who took her to the park near his house for the first time and pushed her on the swings and bounced on the seesaw with her. She mimicked him and often we'd see her walk with her hands behind her back just as he did. The sight of these two beings with similar shaped heads walking to and from the park, lost in conversation with their hands behind their backs was the cutest portrait of the camaraderie between grandparent and grandchild.

She was barely two years old when she began gardening (really pottering in the garden) with grandpa. He gave her a small garden fork, spade and a little bucket and she'd be out in her khaki or maroon overalls digging. They spent ages out there, though I can't say she learned much in the way of planting, pruning or digging because — not without excessive bribery — have I been able to get her to lift a finger to plant tiny herbs let alone plants. I think gardening was something special she did with grandpa and it wasn't so much about plants as it was about cultivating their bond and enriching the soil of their strongly rooted relationship.

During summer trips to the beach, dad spent hours building sandcastles with her; they would also dig huge holes which he got into and then he'd let her cover him with sand. You'd hear their laughter ring across the shoreline as she poured water and sand over him. Mum and I both have a healthy respect for the sea — as well as a deep-seated fear. So it was dad who frolicked in the ocean with his granddaughter, holding her hands as they jumped over the waves. Even as recently as last year, she was still laughing with grandpa as they raced the waves on Noosa beach in Queensland.

Many years before, not long after her second birthday, my daughter became very ill with salmonella poisoning and ended up isolated in a private hospital room. I didn't sleep for three solid nights, so those days are somewhat vague for me. Though I was confined to that hospital room with her, I remember not much more than her high pitched screams from the pain, copious amounts of poop nappies and throw-ups to pass the time.

When mum and dad were allowed in, dad was often able to soothe her screams with gentle massages on her tummy. He'd often pace the floor with her in his arms until she settled down and fell asleep. And then he'd turn to me and massage my neck and back. Not many words were spoken during that time. I was half insane with worry, delirious from lack of sleep and at times I'd just cry. Dad wouldn't say much just continue soothing out the tension with massages. Mum got me through with home-cooking and ensuring I had a shower daily. Dad got me through by soothing me and the baby with his nurturing touch.

When she was four years old I decided to move to the United States. I'd had a hankering for America for as long as I could remember. One of my closest friends had returned to her native California with her husband and family. My best Aussie male friend had also moved there to work. And I was in search of adventure, reconnections with friends who understood me and love. So I packed up and we left for California.

One of the few times I ever saw my dad cry was the day we flew out from Melbourne airport headed to California in June 2002. Everyone in my family was sad, but it was dad's tears I carried on the fifteen-hour flight. As he went to hug us both and promptly burst into tears, he hung onto her and me in a great bear hug. Was I doing the right thing? I was plagued with the thought because I knew how much he was going to miss his grandchild (probably me too).

I really felt him not wanting to let go, yet doing exactly that. He knew I had to figure things out for myself and pursue a dream even if he didn't understand it. I also knew he was her only father figure until then. She had no idea what was going on and didn't understand we were going away for a long time, possibly for always. But distance didn't break the familial bonds. We spoke weekly to my parents and she continued to grow up with her grandparents through long phone calls.

One Sunday evening she and grandpa were on the phone and he started spluttering, with a very dry cough. Dad had been a smoker since he was eleven and no amount of coaxing, pleading and lecturing about the dangers of smoking made any difference. He refused to give up. But that night, dad's coughing fit on the phone led his granddaughter asking him to stop smoking; she didn't want him to hurt his lungs and body anymore. Mum says he quit the next day and has not had another cigarette since.

Our return to Melbourne two years later, when she was six, reignited and strengthened the pa and 'm'angel' bond. When she's struggled in maths at school, dad's been the one who's tutored her, helped her with her times' tables. He's instilled in her the same respect for reading, learning and education as he did in us. He and mum have attended every school play, sports day, concert and festive event from the time she began grade one to now. She often spends part of her school holidays with her grandparents and she and dad spend hours playing sudoku and doing crosswords. And it's been dad who's taught her to play dominoes and card games. They both hate losing but he doesn't give an inch and has helped her become good at games. They argue over who gets the last serve of mum's home cooking and laugh over the fact that they both love their food so much.

She's hung off dad's every word much the same way I did as a little girl. They watch Aussie rules football together and he loves taunting her as much as she loves taunting him when either of their teams(dad barracks for St Kilda and she's an Essendon fan) are ahead in the league.

Dad's a lot softer on her than he ever was on us. He will discipline her with a stern voice or firm lecture if she gets out of line, but for the most part he spoils her. And the words 'I love you' have come out of his mouth more times in the thirteen years of her life than they ever did in the years preceding that. Through their amazing bond and connection they have both learned that 'the best love is the love you give' and it's not only grandpa who's done the telling. She has too.

Woman

Woman I know you understand
The little child inside the man,
Please remember my life is in your hands,
And woman hold me close to your heart,
However, distant don't keep us apart,
After all it is written in the stars.

('Woman' — *John Lennon*)

'What are you on about, woman?' was a regular phrase from dad's mouth in the early years of his and mum's marriage. When I was very young, I used to wonder if my mum's name *was* 'woman', especially when he was irritated and sometimes simply to annoy her. I can't think of too many occasions when he used that word in an endearing way. Yet I know that he wouldn't have made it through many of his challenges without mum in his life.

In the early years of their married life my parents fought a great deal — mostly about money and how it was spent, but also about family and household structure. Mum was quite submissive and soft-hearted so she didn't oppose dad much; in fact, she did whatever she could to keep the peace and keep his temper in check, often at her own expense. I used to watch her as a child and there were times I didn't understand why she let dad have his way so much, especially when I could clearly see she wasn't happy about a certain decision or experience.

Once, though, when we were young, she did leave and took us kids with her to her mother's house. Grandma promptly told her she'd made her choice and had to live with it and sent us back to dad. Mum didn't leave again after that. Still, I had times in my teen years when I wanted to throttle her for putting up with dad's ill temper, and his tight controls over money. I thought she was too soft and needed to stand up for herself. Now, as the years have gone by and I've matured into a woman and made mistakes through ill-chosen partners, lack of maturity and not understanding what love is really all about, I've grown to see my mum in a very different light.

She's been the still waters that flowed steadily and consistently over dad's rocky exterior and chipped away at the hardness to slowly and steadily encourage the gentler parts of him. Her unwavering love, consistent encouragement and faith have kept him centred in the truth of who he is. Like most women she spent years trying to change him while still loving and nurturing him through every flaw, every challenge and every setback in his life. She would often say that God sent her to dad because he knew no-one else would put up with him. (I believe now that there was some truth in those words.) I don't know that anyone other than my mum with her capacity to love, heart as big as a blue whale's and patience as limitless as the sky could have been suited for my dad. She's been the rock against which my father broke the tide of his emotions, uncertainty and inner conflict.

My mum brought to my dad what he'd not really known as a toddler, young boy and teen — she brought him nurturing. There were times in his life he couldn't recognise or even appreciate it, but it's been this that's held him together like super glue.

Mum understood dad's love affair with good food and made it her mission to ensure he's well fed and nourished with amazing home cooked meals.

Dad's often been flippant about their relationship, joking that he's been imprisoned in marriage longer than Nelson Mandela was imprisoned on Robben Island. But there are rare occasions when he's been romantic, bought her flowers or gifts on special occasions. He will, though, say that he did it to shock her into a heart attack, but she's tough and won't keel over. But when she responds with appreciation and tenderness he glows. He'll not admit it easily, but he has been at his most content when mum's happy.

Around the time of their thirtieth wedding anniversary, they went to South Africa on holiday. Dad organised a special vow renewal ceremony and bought mum the set of pearls (a necklace, bracelet and ring) she'd hankered after for many years. As I've watched my parents' marriage change from highly volatile to (mostly) quiet contentment I know it comes with years of working at it, of navigating the changes that occur not only in the individual personalities, but in the dynamic of the relationship. I know that they've only gotten there because mum never ever gave up on dad. In many ways it is she who has loved and nurtured him into the man he is today. She's indeed been the great woman behind the good man.

I know that as dad faces his challenges with cancer, it is mum who will live through the day-to-day grind of not so good days, fears and possibly tears with dad. I know that it's her home cooking he'll want more than any other food offered to him by well-wishers. I know it's the loving touch of her hands he's going to need to soothe his brow.

Dad has never been short of a word, but for the most part he's conversed from the intellect. Yet, since being diagnosed, I've noticed dad is speaking more emotionally. He's opening up more. But I suspect only mum will really get the raw and gritty truth of his fears and anxieties. He'll still put on a partially brave face for his children, his grandchild and his extended community. Only mum will be the totally safe haven where he'll find respite for she has, after all been the 'woman who understands the little child inside the man' and she has held that child close to her heart these many years, writing their love story in the stars.

Lean on me

Sometimes in our lives we all have pain
We all have sorrow
But if we are wise
We know that there's always tomorrow
Lean on me, when you're not strong
And I'll be your friend
I'll help you carry on
For it won't be long
'Til I'm gonna need
Somebody to lean on

('Lean on Me' — *Bill Withers*)

Not long after dad was diagnosed with cancer, mum, dad, my two sisters and I went to a Body, Mind and Spirit fair to support friends who were involved in the fundraising component of the event.

I hadn't had a psychic reading in a long time and since they were in full supply I decided I'd see what energies were floating around me. The reader was young, vibrant, with a bright smile, and I'd barely sat down when she started talking to me about an illness in my family. She was adamant that I wasn't to be afraid — it had come for reasons other than just ill health or stress in the body. The person who was ill, she said, was long overdue for receiving and that the illness had come to help them receive. I went away from that reading with a bunch of thoughts but mostly realising that it was, indeed, dad's time for receiving.

He has always found it very difficult to receive anything — gifts, money, affection and nurturing. His granddaughter is the only one he's comfortably accepted love, hugs and affection from. When I've wanted to take my parents away with us on holidays I've had to book and pay for the trip first before sharing it with them because I knew if I mentioned it to dad before it was paid for, he'd be discouraging me from spending money on them. I think the only reason he'd ever capitulate to being presented with a paid-for airline ticket was because he hates wasting money more than he hates spending it.

I think dad's equated receiving with vulnerability and obligation. He would rather muddle through or go without, than ask for a handout or help. He's a fiercely proud man, especially of the fact that he's always been able to take care of his family. He raised all of us to be as independent as he's been over the years. We've all benefited from that, but we've also suffered from taking the 'I don't need anyone, I can make it through on my own' approach in life.

My brothers haven't always been forthcoming through their times of challenge and trouble and we've often found out about some of the more trying times in their lives long after the fact. Granted, support in our family has often become blurred and turned into interference, but the intentions of goodwill and well wishing have always been the underlying motivation.

My sisters and I have lamented our challenges with men through the years over glasses of wine, way too much chocolate, cheesecake, other comfort food and soppy girlie movies. We're headstrong and feisty — all three of us — and we've always supported ourselves from the time we began working in our teens. We've tackled most household chores on our own, including the ones men usually do. If we couldn't do the 'men's work', we'd either help each other out, get dad's help or pay for outside help. We've all recently realised that perhaps that's been one of the reasons we've not been successful in our relationships with men in the past. We were too busy being self sufficient and overly independent to allow the guys to contribute to us. We'd taken on dad's MO of not relying too much or too long on anyone,. I have come to realise that everyone likes to feel needed, otherwise why would they want to hang around?

Since dad's cancer diagnosis I've noticed a slight shift in dad and in some of us with regards to our 'super self-sufficient' personas. We're becoming better at receiving and better at leaning on each other and our friends.

For the first time, dad's children and grandchild got to experience the joy of giving to him, without a lecture or reprimand, when we pooled our money and bought him an iPod. He wanted to start listening to meditations and relaxing music to bring more calm and peace into his life. He accepted the gift with a huge smile. 'Thank you', was all he said. And while it was wonderful to see the joy on his face at receiving, it was even more wonderful to feel the joy of being able to give him something so easily and so freely.

This has been a time for interesting emotional responses. The week after dad was diagnosed with cancer I experienced an interesting moment with my boyfriend. My head had been foggy the entire week and my thoughts were scattered. I felt like an emotional wreck, anxious with worry and fearful of what lay ahead for dad. As I reversed my car out of the driveway one afternoon, I hit the fence with the front bumper bar and no matter which way I drove next, I was going to rip the bumper bar. It was the last straw in a very stressful week and I howled like a baby.

My boyfriend happened to call a few moments later and, for once, I didn't pull myself together or switch to the 'superwoman' persona. I continued to sob on the phone. I don't know what I expected from him, but what I got was dinner being picked up, loads of hugs and an evening of nurturing. And I was the better for it the next day. Sometimes when we're hell bent on being super-efficient, super-reliable and super-strong in every area of life, we don't allow others the opportunity to give something of themselves or their time to us.

Dad's always been reliable, efficient and responsible; they're wonderful qualities that have served his family very well. His consistency enveloped us in a feeling of trust. But he has often gone so far above and beyond the norm that at times he appeared super human and with that came the feeling that he didn't need anyone. I now understand how hard that can be for loved ones to deal with sometimes, because they'll often feel like they have nothing to offer or contribute. When I wanted to do things for dad and mum over the years, and he didn't just receive it graciously, I'd find myself teary and upset. I always knew he didn't really need what I wanted to give, but I wanted to give it to him anyway, sometimes just because I wanted to.

Every one of us has leant on dad at various times in our lives — whether for some sage advice, helping us move house, counselling us on business and accounting structures, discussing professional opportunities, babysitting duties… and so much more. It has been a long while before he's truly needed someone to lean on. Even if there were times before he certainly never let on.

But that time is here now. I want to know that there are still many more tomorrows so I'm hoping he will allow us to help him carry on and to be the ones he can lean on through the journey ahead.

My Way

For what is a man? What has he got?
If not himself, then he has naught.
To say the things he truly feels
And not the words of one who kneels.
The record shows I took the blows
And did it my way.
Yes, it was my way.

('My way' — *Frank Sinatra*)

Never a truer song was written for dad than 'My way' made famous by the legendary Frank Sinatra. It is also the song I find the hardest to dance to with dad. Because it is the song he wants played at his funeral.

I'm not yet ready to let dad have his way by playing his favourite song at his funeral. In my mind the end is far from near and there are too many things and so many more dances to experience. It's funny how we all know there's no escaping our mortality, yet still we hope we can negotiate on its timing and even its circumstances.

Whilst we might give mortality a fleeting thought every once in a while when we hear of or see stories of death in our own community or on the news, the raw truth is that we hang unto the unrealistic hope that somehow, some way we will escape. We only pay attention to death when it has come too close for comfort and has intruded into our own homes. And few things these days send us into a tailspin around mortality more than the word cancer.

I feel awfully morbid writing this concluding snippet to dad's tribute, but I also cannot escape the inevitable images of illness and death. I dread them. And I do pray that our house will be passed over, that something like a sign of lamb's blood on a doorpost would make it pass over our doors like the angel of death did in Egypt as recounted in the Book of Exodus. And if we are struck by illness, we plead for a cure from whatever God we believe in.

Dad's pure will and propensity to march to his own drum had me thinking — well maybe more wishing — that he'd have some kind of say-so in how he left this life and that it'd be when he was good and ready. Though I may have resented 'his way' of doing things sometimes in his life and our lives, I can't help but wish that this time things could be 'his way' because I know cancer isn't the way he'd choose to see his life come crashing to a hasty conclusion. Dad's the type who'd want to go while in peak physical condition with his mind and faculties intact.

The image of Tristan Ludlow's character in the movie the 'Legends of the Fall' fighting a grizzly bear comes to mind when I think of dad. In the film they appear to become one as they die at each other's hand. The image freeze-frames as the American Indian, One Stab, concludes the story with, 'It was a good death.' I don't know what would constitute a good death for dad; it might have something to do with being out in nature, facing the elements, perhaps even scaling the face of a mountain.

After the first few weeks of dad's diagnosis I know I said all the 'right' things — the clichéd 'there's a reason for everything', 'it's a time to trust' and all the things that I'd always clung to in challenging times. But I also know they all felt like crap when it was someone I loved so dearly. I felt like a fraud and a fake because I've always thought of myself as one with incredible faith, but I can tell you I was definitely not feeling the faith in the first two weeks of May 2010. It was in my darkest moments of despair one night that I had the feeling that I was being given an opportunity to revisit the years of dad's life and find the treasures in it. I didn't really know where to start but noticed that memories of his life came rushing to my mind for days in a row. I'd be driving to and from work and laughing and crying at the same time. And the strongest theme, in every memory snippet, was how much dad has remained true to himself.

William Shakespeare's quote 'to thine own self be true' was one of the first, and often repeated, sayings that dad quoted from the time he first introduced me to the Classics. And I realised he'd taken it on as a subconscious mantra in almost every sphere of his own life.

From the very early years of his life, as the abandoned boy in the orphanage, he found his own way to survive particularly exercising his boyish charm to get the nuns to spoil him and give him what he wanted.

As the teen grew into a man, he found his own way to connect to God and his inner spirit through exploring the rituals of Catholicism and the magnificence of nature. The teasing and ridicule of others never stopped him from finding out what he wanted and needed to know to satisfy his spiritual curiosity. He stopped going to church only when we'd already been living in Australia for a few years and only when he wanted to. And he offered no explanation or apologies to anyone, including God I would guess.

As father and husband he has been upfront about the fact that life is a lot easier for his family if we do what he wants and as he says. The less we opposed dad over the years, the more peaceful it was. Whether it was the 'right' way by other people's standards never entered his mind. It was his way.

As a professional man, who followed his own work ethic, his focus was always on doing his personal best. He was driven by his personal values regardless if they aligned with anyone else or not. And he won and reciprocated respect from the wealthiest executive in the plush office suites to the lowest paid labourer in the quarry.

The philanthropist and humanitarian in him saw him contribute his time and energy to causes that may have been viewed as a 'waste of time' or not worth pursuing since they may not have yielded quick results if any at all. But dad followed his own heart. If at times that meant he stood alone in his beliefs, so be it. He never wanted to compromise himself.

It is only as a grandpa that I've seen dad bend a little. I've seen the pure love of a curly headed granddaughter with big, dark brown eyes melt his heart and twist him around her little finger. But since they're similar in so many ways, I'm not always sure who's bending to whose will. Perhaps it's their kindred spirits exercising a collective will on the rest of us unsuspecting victims.

I don't know that I'd have paused long enough to dance with the treasures of dad's life if cancer hadn't come knocking on his door. Whilst there are moments I still want to punch it square in the face, I'm clear now why it entered my life via dad. Somehow it doesn't feel quite so frightening anymore.

And I'm grateful that I've been given the opportunity to enjoy these wonderful dances with my father — the dances of an incredible life. Otherwise I'd have been like most other people who get to honour or value someone in a eulogy. What good is that?

I know I would not have wanted to miss the most meaningful legacy of dad's life — that the only true way to live one's life is to 'say the things one truly feels and not the words of one who kneels' and to be proud of the fact that it was always lived 'my way'.

Epilogue

Some months have passed since dad was first diagnosed with prostate cancer. It's been as daunting and as eye-opening as I expected it to be. As a family, we've experienced the full gamut of love, fears, tears, laughter, avoidance, denial and humour.

One of the highlights of the journey so far was a moment of uncontained laughter I shared with dad and mum as we watched my daughter's Saturday morning netball game. Dad was filling me in on his discussion with the specialist about having prostate surgery. He was given the option of keyhole surgery but when asked to describe his body type and weight over the phone, the specialist replied that his circumference around the waist might be too big for keyhole surgery. Dad ended the story by saying, 'Well it seems I'm too fat for this keyhole surgery. Looks like my paunch has finally tripped me up,' and hooted with laughter. He, mum and I laughed so hard we nearly fell onto the netball court. It was great to have tears of laughter streaming down my face rather than those of fear and sadness.

A few weeks later I paced a hospital floor, edgy and irate because dad was still not down from surgery and none of the nurses could tell us why. We'd expected him to be out of surgery after four to five hours, but after six hours there was no sign of him and it didn't matter who we tried to talk to, they were not divulging any information. The 'not knowing' drove me crazy and I'm ashamed to admit it but I got rather forceful with one of the nurses and reminded her there was a very worried family waiting around.

She eventually did find the nurse assigned to dad and we were told he was out of surgery and would be returning to the ward soon. Soon turned out to be another thirty or so minutes and by then I was ready to climb the walls. When they brought him back to the ward I wanted to vanish into thin air. I've never seen dad look so fragile. He was heavily sedated, incoherent and looked like a helpless little boy. It was really, really hard to see him so frail. It was in that moment I realised that this experience with cancer wasn't all that different to any of life's experiences. One moment you're up and in the throes of belly laughter; the next you're weighed down by unspoken fear and anxiety.

The thing about cancer is that it intensifies the experiences, probably because it carries a sledge hammer of doom. And perhaps its only gift, like all other terminal illnesses, is that once it comes knocking it not only raises the awareness of death, but also the awareness of life. Though I've read one of my favourite books *Tuesdays with Morrie,* by Mitch Albom, many times over it has become a source of solace and deep comfort to me over the last months. And I think I finally understand what Morrie was trying to teach Mitch when he said:

'The truth is, Mitch, once you learn how to die, you learn how to live… Most of us walk around as if we're sleepwalking. We really don't experience the world fully because we're half asleep, doing things we automatically think we have to do… Learn how to die, and you learn how to live.'

I'm hoping that all those on the journey of cancer and other terminal illnesses will learn more about dying so we can get better at living.

Follow me at my blog;   www.waalexander.com